ANTI BACTERIAL ACTIVITY OF TUKHM-E-MOOLI

(SEED OF *RAPHANUS SATIVUS LINN.*)

Regd. No. 24/8/10

Dissertation submitted to Dr. NTR University of Health Sciences,

Vijayawada, A.P. for award of the degree of

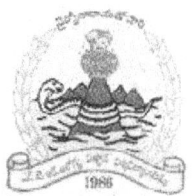

DOCTOR OF MEDICINE

IN

ILMUL ADVIA (Pharmacology)

BY

FAIYAZ AHMAD

B.Sc., BUMS (ALLD)

POST GRADUATE DEPARTMENT OF ILMUL ADVIA

(PHARMACOLOGY)

GOVT.NIZAMIA TIBBI COLLEGE

CHARMINAR, HYDERABAD.

2012

CERTIFICATE

This is certified that Faiyaz Ahmad a bonafied P.G .Scholar, Department of Ilmul Advia (pharmacology), Govt. Nizamia Tibbi College Charminar, Hyderabad, affiliated to Dr. NTR University of Health Sciences, Vijayawada, A.P, India.

He has carried out research work entitled **"ANTIBACTERIALACTIVITY OF TUKHM-E-MOOLI (SEED OF *RAPHANUS SATIVUS LINN.*)."**

Under supervision and guidance of Dr. Abdul Saleem, Assist. Professor P.G. Dept.of ILMUL-ADVIA Govt. Nizamia Tibbi College Charminar, Hyderabad.

Prof. Dr.Wasia Naveed
M.D
Principal
Govt. NizamiaTibbi College
Charminar, Hyderabad, A.P

ENDORSEMENT BY THE HEAD OF THE DEPARTMENT

This is to certify that Faiyaz Ahmad, a bonafied P.G .Scholar, Department of Ilmul Advia (Pharmacology), Govt. Nizamia Tibbi College, Charminar, Hyderabad, affiliated to Dr. NTR University of Health Sciences, Vijayawada, A.P, India.

He has carried out research work entitled **"ANTIBACTERIALACTIVITY OF TUKHM-E-MOOLI (SEED OF *RAPHANUS SATIVUS LINN.*),"** Under supervision and guidance of Dr. Abdul Saleem Assist. Professor, Dept. of ILMUL-ADVIA Govt. Nizamia Tibbi College Charminar, Hyderabad.

Prof. Dr. Mir Yousuf Ali
B.Sc (Hons.) M.D (UHS)
P.G. Prof. & HOD
P.G. Dept. of ILMUL-ADVIA
Govt. Nizamia Tibbi College
Charminar, Hyderabad, A.P

CERTIFICATE

This is to certify that Faiyaz Ahmad, a bonafied P.G .Scholar, Department of Ilmul Advia (pharmacology), Govt. Nizamia Tibbi College, Charminar, Hyderabad, affiliated to Dr. NTR University of Health Sciences, Vijayawada, A.P, India

He has carried out his research work entitled **"ANTIBACTERIAL ACTIVITY OF TUKHM-E-MOOLI (SEED OF *RAPHANUS SATIVUS LINN.*)."** Under supervision and guidance of the regulations laid down by the Dr. NTR University of Health sciences, for the award of the Degree of DOCTOR of MEDICINE in the specialty of Ilmul Advia (Pharmacology).

Co-Guide   **Guide**

Ayesha Mateen   **Dr. Abdul Saleem**
M.Sc. (Microbiology)   M.D. (UHS)
SRF, Dept. of Pharmacognosy   Assist. Professor CRIUM,
Erragadda, Hyderabad   P.G. Dept. of ILMUL-ADVIA
                                                       Govt. Nizamia Tibbi College
                                                       Charminar, Hyderabad

CENTRAL RESEARCH INSTITUTE OF UNANI MEDICINE

(AN ISO 9001:2000 CERTIFIED INSTITUTE)

 केन्द्रीय यूनानी चिकित्सा अनुसंधान संस्थान

కేంద్రీయ యూనానీ వైద్య పరిశోధన సంస్థ مرکزی تحقیقاتی ادارہ برائے طب یونانی

(Central Council for Research in Unani Medicine, New Delhi - Under Ministry of Health & F.W., Govt. of India)

8-3-168/A/1/UM, A G's Colony Road, Erragadda, Hyderabad - 500 038, (A.P.) India
☎ Director : 23811551 Fax : 040-23811495 Off : 23810246 E-mail : criumhyderabad@yahoo.com

F.No.19-10/2011-CRIUM/Tech/   Dated:24.03.2012

TO WHOM SO EVER IT MAY CONCERN

This is to certify that as part of his M.D. thesis, **Dr. Faiyaz Ahmad**, P.G Scholar, Department of Ilmul-Advia (Pharmacology), Govt. Nizamia Tibbi College, Hyderabad has done studies pertaining to Drug identification, Authentication, Standardization & Antibacterial activity of different extracts of Tukhm-e-Mooli (seeds of *Raphanus sativus*) in this Institute during March to May, 2011. Dr. V.C. Gupta, Deputy Director (Botany), Mrs. Atiya Rehana, Research Officer (Chemistry), Mr. Mohd. Abdul Rasheed, N., SRF (Chemistry) and Ms. Ayesha Mateen, SRF (Microbiology) provided him necessary assistance under the guidance of the Director of the Institute.

(DR. MUSHTAQ AHMAD)
DIRECTOR
Dr. MUSHTAQ AHMAD
M.D.
Director
Central Research Institute of Unani Medicine
Ministry of Health & F.W. Govt. of India.
Erragadda, Hyderabad-038.

DECLARATION

I, Faiyaz Ahmad, post graduate Scholar, P.G. Department of Ilmul-Advia, Govt. Nizamia Tibbi College, Charminar, Hyderabad. Solemnly declare that the research Work done on **"ANTIBACTERIAL ACTIVITY OF TUKHM-E-MOOLI (SEED OF *RAPHANUS SATIVUS LINN.*)."** during the period, 2009-2012 is absolutely a bonafide and genuine work.

Faiyaz Ahmad

B.Sc., BUMS
P.G. Scholar
P.G. Dept. of Ilmul-Advia
Govt. Nizamia Tibbi College
Charminar, Hyderabad.

DEDICATED
TO
MY

Mother Land
Ballia

&

Home Land
Yusufpur

ACKNOWLEDGMENT

I first thank Almighty ALLAH the most beneficent and merciful for providing me an opportunity to complete this work.

I am very grateful to my respected, honorable and beloved parents Janab **Anwar Ali Ansari** & Mohtrema **Nadira Khatoon**, who encouraged me constantly, without their blessing, support and affection this study could not have been completed.

I would like to thank Prof. Dr. Wasia Naveed, Principal and HoD, Department of Amraz-e-Niswa wa Qabalat, GNTC, Charminar, Hyderabad.

I express my gratitude to Prof. Dr. Mir Yousuf Ali, MD, Head of the P.G. Department of ILMUL ADVIA (Pharmacology), Govt. Nizamia Tibbi College Charminar, Hyderabad, A.P., for his advice throughout my studies.

I am very grateful to my Guide Dr. Abdul Saleem Assist. Professor, Department of ILMUL ADVIA (Pharmacology), GNTC who helped me to a great extends in my research work. I am thankful to him for his guidance, valuable suggestion, help and co-operation throughout my studies.

My extreme thanks to my Co-Guide Mrs. Ayesha Mateen, SRF (Microbiology) CRIUM (Erragadda) for her suggestion, guidance and help throughout my dissertation work. She has been very kind and cooperative throughout my Experimental work.

I am very thankful to Dr. Md. Mohsin MD, Lecturer, and Dr. Noor Banu Noorien MD for their kind help and cooperation during my dissertation work.

I am also thankful to Dr. Mushtaq Ahmad, Director, CRIUM, for granting me permission to conduct some part of my experimental work in their institute.

I am thankful to Mr. M.A. Rasheed N., SRF (Chemistry), Mrs. Atiya Rehana SSA (Chemistry), DSRU In-charge and Mr. Ahmad (Office Boy) for their kind help and co-operation.

I would like to thank Dr. V.C. Gupta, Deputy Director (Botany), CRIUM, for identification and authentication of drug.

I am immensely thankful to librarians and staff of GNTC, CRIUM, Salarjung Museum for their cooperation, and help to providing me needful material during my dissertation work.

I would like to express my wholehearted thanks and gratitude to my all the teachers of State Unani Medical College (SUMC), Allahabad, Specially Dr. Saad Usmani, Ex-Principal, SUMC, Allahabad, Dr. Mohd. Sikandar Hayat, Director,Unani Medical Services, Govt. of Utter Pradesh, Lucknow, U.P. Dr. Mohd Mazahir Alam, Principal, SUMC, Allahabad and Dr. Mohammad Hasan, M.O. SUMC Allahabad. Who were a constant source of inspiration, encouragement & goal suggestion throughout the course of the study.

I convey my special thanks to my seniors, colleagues and juniors of Ilmul Advia Dept. GNTC, Hyd. for their support in the completion of this work.

I am especially thankful to my good friend Syed Azizullah Hussainy R. of Chennai, P.G. Scholar, Dept. of Kulliyat-e-Tib, GNTC for his co-operation and being a constant source of inspiration for me.

I would like to thank my spiritual teacher Hazarat Maulana Suhail Ahmad of Bahadurganj, Ghazipur, U.P. Ustad-e-Fiqh, Darul Uloom Rahmania, Hyderabad for his support, guidance and co-operation and being a constant source of inspiration for me.

Finally I would like to thank everybody who has helped me to the successful realization of this dissertation.

Faiyaz Ahmad

ABSTRACT

ANTIBACTERIAL ACTIVITY OF TUKHM-E-MOOLI
(SEED OF *RAPHANUS SATIVUS* L.)

Raphanus sativus L. (Radish) is an annual herb of family Cruciferae and grown as an edible root.

Objectives: The aim of the study is to test the potentiality of the drug in different solvent extracts (Ethanol, Methanol, Ethyl Acetate, Chloroform, Benzene, Aqueous hot and Aqueous cold) against various pathogenic bacterial strains *E.coli* (ATCC-25922), *Klebsiella pneumonia* (ATCC-27736), *Proteus vulgaris (ATCC-6380), Pseudomonas aeruginosa* (ATCC-27853), *Staphylococcus aureus* (ATCC-25923), *Shigella sonnie* (ATCC-25931), *Salmonella typhi* (ATCC-25241) and *Salmonella paratyphi* (ATCC-9150), and to determine the antibacterial activity.

Methods: The antibacterial activity was performed in vitro using Agar well diffusion assay and diameter of zone of inhibition was measured.

Results: Among all the extracts of the test drug the Ethanolic and Methanolic extracts showed maximum antibacterial activity against all the bacterial strain used with a zone of inhibition ranges from 12-21mm and the least activity was observed in Aqueous cold extract with zone of inhibition ranges from 7-9mm. The test results were compared with standard antibiotics chloramphenicol and Ciprofloxacin.

Conclusions: The qualitative analysis of different extracts of *Raphanus sativus* seed reveals the presence of Alkaloids, Flavonoids, Glycosides, Phenols, Tannins, Saponin, Sterols and Protein which may be responsible for the observed antibacterial activity. The results suggest that ethanolic and methanolic extracts can be used in the treatment of infection caused by these bacterial strains used in this study.

Key words: Antibacterial Activity, Phytochemical Analysis, *Raphanus sativus,* Zone of Inhibition

ABBREVIATIONS

WHO	-	World Health Organization
B.C	-	Before Christ
A.D.	-	After the Death of Christ
Ex.eg	-	Example
μm	-	Micrometer
-ve	-	Negative
+ve	-	positive
CF	-	Ciprofloxacin
Mm	-	Millimeter
Ft	-	Feet
Mt	-	Methanolic extract
Et	-	Ethanol extract
Ea	-	Ethyl acetate
Ch	-	Chloroform
Ben	-	Benzene
Aq	-	Aqueous
Gm	-	Gram
Mg	-	Milligram
μlt	-	Micro liter
ZOI	-	Zone of inhibition
TLC	-	Thin Layer Chromatography
HPTLC	-	High Performance Thin Layer Chromatography
ATCC	-	American Type of Culture Collection

CONTENTS

TOPICS   PAGE NO.

PART I

S.NO.   **LITERATURE REVIEW**

PART II
EXPERIMENTAL STUDY

PART III

PART - I

INTRODUCTION

Serious infections caused by bacteria that have become resistant to commonly used antibiotic have become a major global health care problem in the 21st century. In the developing countries bacterial infections are still the main cause of the death [1]. According to World Health Organization (WHO), the increase of resistance to antibiotics by bacterial pathogens is a growing problem in both developed and developing countries.[2,3] Antimicrobial resistance is a natural biological phenomenon exacerbated by the misuse of drugs.[4,5] According to World Health Organization (WHO), the increase of resistance to antibiotics by bacterial pathogens is a growing problem in both developed and developing countries.[2,3] Antibacterial resistance is a natural biological phenomenon exacerbated by the misuse of drugs.[4,5] Occurrence of multidrug resistant pathogens is ever increasing, and the treatment of such strains has led to the administration of very large doses of antibiotics, resulting in enormous ammount of side effects to the patients.[3, 6] The problem of microbial resistance is growing and the outlook of the use of antimicrobial drugs in future is uncertain. Therefore action must be taken to reduce this problem, for example, to control the use of antibiotics, to develop research to better understanding of the genetic mechanism of resistance and to continue study to develop new drugs either synthetic or natural.[4,7] Natural resources, especially the plants are the potent condidates for this purpose.

Plants play important role in our daily life. They not only provide us nutrition but also play a significant role in providing medicine. Medicinal plants have served humans through ages as a constant source of medicament for the treatment of a variety of diseases. Plants are used medicinally in different countries and are a source of many potent and powerful drugs. Different parts of plants, herbs and spices have been used for many years for the prevention of infection.[4,8] Medicinal plants represent a rich source of antimicrobial agent. The use of plants with known antimicrobial properties can be of great significance in treatment of infections.[4,7,9] A renewed interest in plant based antimicrobials has arisen during the last twenty years, but still plant based antimicrobials are poorly explored. Screening of plants extracts for antimicrobial activity has shown that higher plants represent a potential source of new anti-infective compounds.[10] The antimicrobial compounds from plants may inhibit bacteria through different mechanism than the conventional antibiotics, and could therefore be of clinical value in the treatment of microbial infection.[11] The primary benefits of using plant-derived medicines are that they are relatively safer than synthetic antibiotics, offering profound therapeutic benefits and more affordable treatment.[12,13]

Only a small fraction of the known plant species of the whole world have been evaluated for the presence of antimicrobial compounds, and thus it is necessary to increase the efforts in collecting and screening plants for the development of novel and environmentally safe antimicrobial agents.[14]

Radish, *Raphanus sativus* Linn. (Brassicaceae family) is an annual herb, consumed as vegetable, commonly known as Mooli. It is coarse, rough or glabrous. Leaves are lyrate, pinnate or pinnatifid. Flowers are large yellow, white or pale lilac, veined with purple, in long ebracteate racemes. Seeds are pendulous, globose; cotyledons conduplicate. It is cultivated all over sub-continent up to 16,000 ft in temperate and warm countries.[15] It is well reputed in Unani System of Medicine, useful for urinary complaints and piles. Almost all parts of the plant including leaves, seeds and roots are utilized in medicine. The fresh juices obtained from leaves are diuretic, laxative. Roots are used for urinary complaints and syphilitic disease; they are a reputed medicine for piles and gastrodynic pains. The seeds are peptic, expectorant, diuretic, laxative, carminative, antitussive and stomach tonic.[15, 16, 17, 18]

In the view of this, the present study aims at assessing the antibacterial property of *R. sativus* seed extract, and to substantiate the use of radish in unani system of medicine in infectious diseases.

THE UNANI PERSPECTIVE OF BACTERIOLOGY

The Unani System of Medicine is a time tested medicine based on Hypothesis, Experience and Investigations. The ancient Unani physicians hypothesized the concept of Ajsam-e- khabisah (microorganism), Ta'diyah (Infection), and Ufunat (Putrefaction) in their ways.[19]

The Great Medical Scholar of 9th century **Al-Razi** was aware of air born infections. He proved his philosophy of microbes, infections and Putrefaction through his thought and experiment. He was the Medical Director of a great hospital in Baghdad. When he asked regarding the selection of site for construction of a new hospital in Baghdad. He experimented the philosophy of microbes and infections by hanging a piece of meat in the air of different places and noticed that where it putrefied soon due to the air born infection / Putrefaction. Hence he decided to construct the new hospital, at the place where the Putrefaction takes place durably (because of least presence of microbes and infection). Al Razi wrote the first medical description of Small pox and Measles and described the clinical differences between two diseases so vividly that nothing since has been added, in his famous Book Kitab-al-Judri wal Hisbah (The Book of Small pox and Measles).[20] **Ali ibn Abbas Majoosi** described contagious diseases like leprosy, elephantiasis.[21]

Abu Ali Ibn Sina (Avicenna, 980-1037) stated explicitly that water did not putrefied alone, until it mixed up with Ajsam-e-arzia khabisah (earthy microbes) and after that raddi kaifiyet (bad quality) developed. The Putrefaction of air also takes place in same way.[22, 23, 24, 25]

He also hypothesized on the contagious nature of Tuberculosis and other infectious diseases, and used quarantine as a means of limiting the spread of contagious diseases.[26]

Ibn Khatima (1369 AD) was the first to observed that mankind is surrounded by Ghair maryee (non visible) Ajsam-e-saghirah (minute bodies) and also described that how minute bodies enter into the human body and cause disease well in-advance of Pasteur's discovery of microbes. There is a famous story about Ibn Khatima, once he fell ill, being a physician he tried to find out the cause of his illness. But he did not find any exact cause of his illness. Then he realized that some non-visible tiny bodies were entering into his body through respiratory tract while he used to refer the old wicked books. These minute bodies are real cause of his illness.[24]

Ibn Al-Khatib (1313 – 1374/5) was the first who explained the existence of contiguity in detail. He composed a treatise in the defence of the theory of Infection in following way: To those who say, "How can we admit the possibility of infection while the religious low denies it?" we reply that "The existence of contagion is established by experience, investigation, the evidence of the senses and trustworthy reports. These facts constitute a sound argument. The fact of infection becomes clear to the investigator who notices how he who establishes contact with the afflicted gets the disease, whereas he who is not in contact remains safe, and how transmission is affected through garments, vessels and earrings.[26]

Abu Mansoor-Al Hasan bin Nooh-Al Qamari in "**Ghina wa Muna**" discovered the cause and effect of Gonorrhoea century before it was documented by the Europeans.[27]

These passages seems to indicate that the Unani Physician were aware of the existence of microorganisms, their infectious and communicable properties. But there were lack of facilities and experimental instruments, through which their philosophies and theories can be interpreted.

MICROBIOLOGY

Microbiology is the branch of science that deals with microorganisms. Micro means very small and biology is the study of living things, so microbiology is the study of very small living things normally too small to be seen with the naked eye.[29] Microbiology has become an umbrella term that encompasses many sub disciplines or fields of study. These include Bacteriology,Mycology, Protozoology, Phycology, Parasitological, and Virology.[29]

History of Microbiology:

The existence of microorganisms was hypothesized from many centuries before their actual discovery .**Varo and Columella** in the first century B.C. postulated that diseases were caused by invisible beings. **Fracastorius** (1546) proposed a 'Contagium vivum' as a possible cause of infectious disease.[30]**Antonie van Leeuwenhoek** (1632-1723), a draper observed bacteria and other microorganisms, using a single-lens microscope of his own design and called them 'Little Animalcules'. The earliest discovery of a pathogenic microorganism was probably made by **Agostino Bassi** (1835), who showed that the muscardine disease of silk worm was caused by a fungus. **Davaine & Pollender** (1850) observed anthrax bacilli in the blood of animal dying of the disease. In fact, even before microbial cause of infections had been established, **Oliver Wendell Holmes** in the USA (1843) and **Ignaz**

Semmelweis in Vienna (1846) had independently concluded that puerperal sepsis was contagious. Semmelweis also identified its mode of transmission by doctors and medical students attending on women in labour in the hospital and had prevented it by the simple measures of washing of hands in an antiseptic solution, for which service to medicine and humanity, he was persecuted by medical orthodoxy and driven insane.[30] **Louis Pasteur** (1822-95) is a founder of "germ theory of disease" as he visualized that diseases are caused by microorganisms. He has also described the process of Fermentation and Pasteurization. He is considered as "father of microbiology", as his contribution led to the development of microbiology as a separate scientific discipline. **Robert Koch** (1843-1910) perfected bacteriological technique. He introduced staining techniques and method of obtaining bacteria in pure culture using solid media. Koch is best known for his contributions to the germ theory of disease, proving that specific diseases were caused by specific pathogenic micro-organisms. He developed a series of criteria that have become known as the **Koch's postulates. Joseph Lister** (1827-1912) successfully prevented post operative sepsis by introducing antiseptic techniques. **Ivanovsky** (1892) reproduced mosaic disease in the tobacco plant by applying to healthy leave juice from the diseased plants from which all bacteria had been removed by passage through fine filters. **Beijerinck** (1898) confirmed these findings and coined the term *virus* for such filterable infectious agents. **Stanley** (1935) was able to obtain the infectious agent of tobacco-mosaic in a crystalline form. **Metchnikoff** (1845-1916) discovered the phenomenon of Phagocytosis and proposed the phagocytic response as the prime defence against the microbial invasion of tissues. **Paul Ehrlich** (1854-1915) pioneered the technique of antimicrobial chemotherapy in medicine. **Flemming** (1881-1955) in 1929 made the accidental discovery that the fungus *Penicillum notatum* produces a substance that destroys *Staphylococcus*. **Macfarlane Burnet** (1957) proposed clonal selection theory to explain antibody synthesis. In 1967 he developed the concept of "immunological Surveillance", according to which the primary function of the immune system is to preserve the integrity of the body, seeking and destroy all foreign antigens, whether autogenous or external in origin.[30, 31, 32, 33]

BACTERIA

Bacteria are prokaryotic microorganisms that don't contain chlorophyll. They are unicellular and don't show true branching, except in the so-called higher bacteria.

Habitat: Bacteria are present in most habitats on earth, growing in soil, acid hot springs, radioactive wastes, water and deep in the earth's crust, as well as in organic matter and the living bodies of plants and animals, and in the digestive tracts of humans.

Morphology of bacteria: Morphologically the bacteria can be differentiated as follows-

i. **Cocci:** These are round or oval bacteria about 0.5-1.0 μm in diameter.

ii. **Bacilli:** These are rod shaped or stick like bacteria about 1-10 μm in length and 0.3-1.0 μm in width.

iii. **Vibrios:** These bacteria are comma shaped, curved rod, measuring about 3-4 μm in length and 0.5 μm in width. Most of them are motile with a single flagellum at one end.

iv. **Spirulla:** These are regularly coiled, rigid organisms, about 3-4 μm in length. These are motile with group of flagella at both ends.

v. **Spirochetes:** These are flexible and motile organisms. They are about 6-15 μm in length and 0.2-0.5 μm in width.

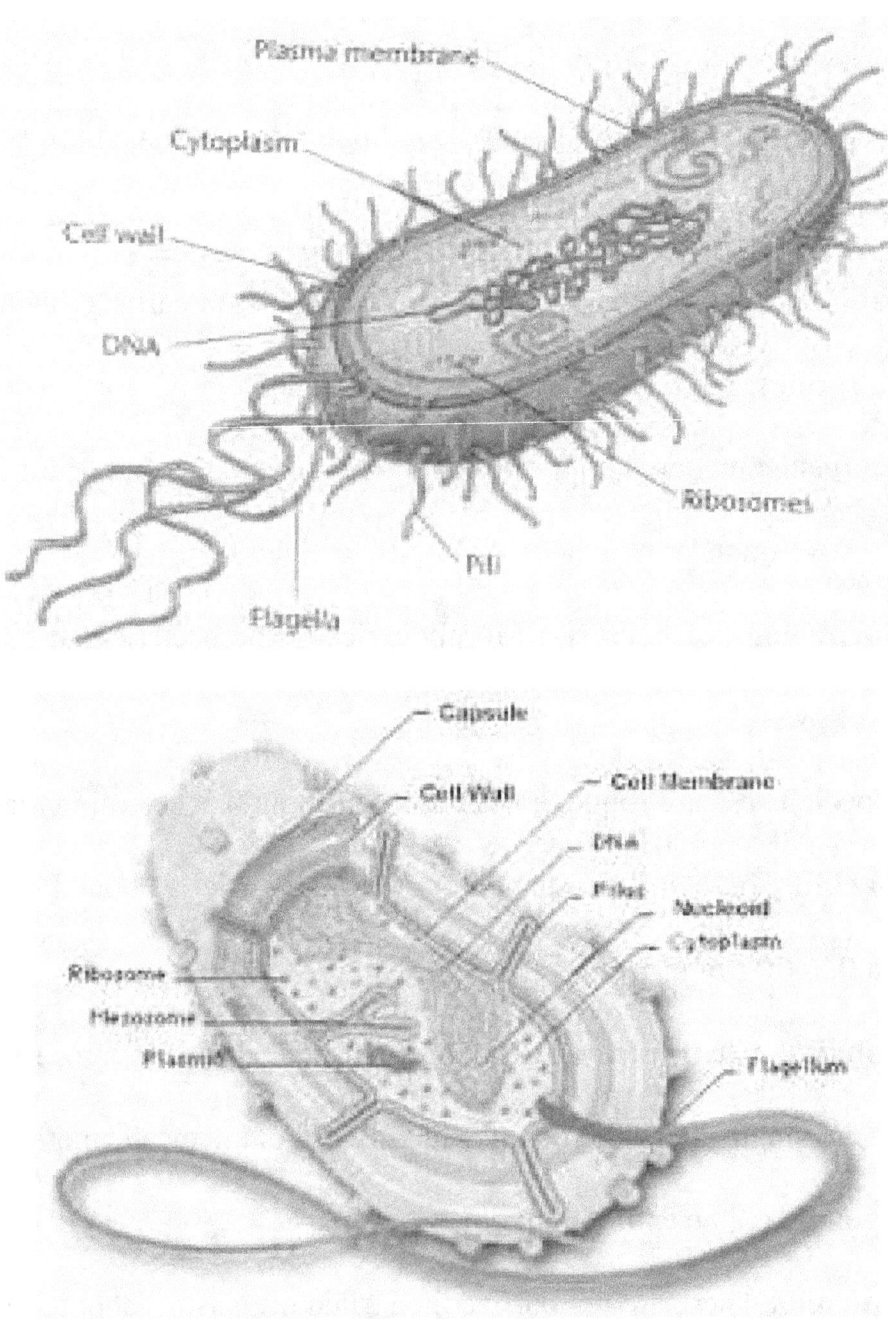

Fig: Structure of bacteria

Bacterial Anatomy: The outer layer or cell envelope consist of two components- a rigid cell wall and beneath it a cytoplasmic or plasma membrane. The cell envelope encloses the protoplasm, comprising the cytoplasm, cytoplasmic inclusions such as ribosomes and mesosomes, granules, vacuoles and the nuclear body. Besides these essential components, some bacteria may possess additional structures. The cell may be enclosed in a viscid layer, which may be loose slime layer, or organized as a capsule. Some bacteria carry filamentous appendages protruding from the cell surface- the flagella which are organs of locomotion and the fimbriae which appear to be organs for adhesion.

Cell wall: The cell wall accounts for the shape of the bacterial cell and confers on it rigidity and ductility. Bacterial cell walls are about 10-25 nm thick and account for about 20-30 percent of the dry weight of the cells. Chemically the cell wall is composed of mucopeptide (peptidoglycan or murein). In general, the walls of gram positive bacteria have a simpler chemical nature than those of gram negative bacteria.

Cytoplasmic membrane: The cytoplasmic (plasma) membrane is a thin (5-10nm) layer lining the inner surface of the cell wall and separating it from the cytoplasm. It acts as a semi permeable membrane controlling the flow of metabolites to and from the protoplasm.

Cytoplasm: The bacterial cytoplasm is a colloidal system of a variety of organic and inorganic solutes in a viscous watery solution. It differs from eukaryotic cytoplasm in not exhibiting internal mobility and in the absence of endoplasmic reticulum or mitochondria. The cytoplasm contains ribosomes, mesosomes, inclusions and vacuoles.

Intracytoplasmic inclusions: Intracytoplasmic inclusions may be of various types, the chief of which are volutin, polysaccharide, lipid and crystal. They are characteristic of different species.

Nucleus: Bacterial nuclei have no nuclear membrane or nucleolus. The nuclear DNA is not associated with basic protein. The genome consist of a single molecule of double-stranded DNA arranged in the form of a circle, which may open under certain condition to form a long chain, about 1 mm in length. The bacterial chromosome is haploid and replicates by simple fission instead of by mitosis in other cell. Bacteria may possess extranuclear genetic elements consisting of DNA. These cytoplasmic carriers of genetic information are termed plasmid or episomes.

Slim layer and capsule: Many bacteria secrete a viscid material around the cell surface. When this is organized into a sharply defined structure, it is known as the capsule. When it is a loose undermarcated secretion, it is called the slime layer. The slime is generally, but not invariably, polysaccharide or poly peptide in nature. Some bacteria may have both a capsule and a slime layer.

Flagella: Motile bacteria, except spirochetes, possess one or more unbranched, long, sinuous filaments called flagella, which are the organ of locomotion. Each flagellum consists of three distinct parts, the filament, the hook and the basal body. The filament is external to the cell and connected to the hook at the cell surface. The flagella are 3-20 μm long and are of uniform diameter (0.01-0.013 μm) and terminate in a square tip. The presence or absence of flagella and their number and arrangement are characteristic of different genera of bacteria.

Fimbriae: Some gram negative bacilli carry very fine, hair-like surface appendages called fimbriae or pili. They are shorter and thinner than flagella (about 0.5 μm long and less than 10 nm thick) and project from the cell surface as straight filaments. They are unrelated to motility and are found on motile as well as non-motile cells. Fimbriae function as organ of adhesion, helping the cell to adhere firmly to particles of various kinds. This property may serve to anchor the bacteria in nutritionally favourable microenvironments.

Spore: Some bacteria, particularly member of the genera bacillus and Clostridium have the ability to form highly resistant resting stages called spores. Each bacterium forms one spore, which on germination forms a single vegetative cell. Sporulation in bacteria, therefore, is not a method of reproduction. As bacterial spores are formed inside the parent cell, they are called endospores.

Pleomorphism and involution forms: Some species of bacteria exhibit great variation in the shape and size of individual cells. This is known as pleomorphism. Certain species show swollen and aberrant forms in ageing culture, especially in the presence of high salt concentration. These are known as involution forms. Many of the cells may be nonviable. Pleomorphism and involution forms are often caused by defective cell wall synthesis. Involution forms may also develop due to the activity of autolytic enzymes.

Bacterial Nutrition: Bacteria can be classified nutritionally, based on their energy requirements and on their ability to synthesis essential metabolites. Bacteria which derived their energy from sunlight are called **phototrophs** (cyanobacteria, green sulferbacteria) and those that obtain energy from chemical reaction are called **chemotrophs** (Bacillus, Clostridium). Bacteria that can synthesis all their organic compounds are called **autotrophs** (cyanobacteria, phototrophic bacteria). Those that are unable to synthesis their own metabolites and depends on performed organic compounds are called **heterotrophs** (helicobacteria, sulphur bacteria). Autotrophs are able to utilize atmospheric carbon dioxide and nitrogen. Heterotrophic bacteria are unable to grow with carbon dioxide as the sole source of carbon. The nutritional requirements of heterotrophs vary widely. Some may require only a single organic substance such as glucose, while others may need a large number of different compounds such as amino acids, nucleotides, lipid, carbohydrates and coenzymes. Bacteria require a supply of inorganic salts, particularly the anions phosphate and sulphate, and the cation sodium, potassium magnesium, iron, manganese and calcium. Some bacteria required certain organic compounds in minute quantities. These are known as growth factors or bacterial vitamins. Growth factors are called essential when growth does not occur in their absence or accessory when they enhance growth, without being absolutely necessary for it.

Metabolism: Depending on the influence of oxygen on growth and viability, bacteria are divided into aerobes and anaerobes. **Anaerobic bacteria** required oxygen for growth. They may be **obligate aerobes** like the *cholera vibrio,* which will grow only in the presence of oxygen, or **facultative anaerobes** which are ordinarily aerobic but can also grow in the absence of oxygen, through less abundantly. Most bacteria of medical importance are facultative anaerobes. Anaerobic bacteria, such as *clostridia*, grow in the absence of oxygen and the **obligate anaerobes** may even die on exposure to oxygen.

Microaerophilic bacteria are those that grow best in the presence of low oxygen tension.

Aerobic bacteria obtain their energy and intermediates only through oxidation, involving oxygen as the ultimate hydrogen acceptor, while the anaerobes use hydrogen acceptors other than oxygen. Facultative anaerobes may act in both ways. A more common process in anaerobic metabolism may be a series of oxidoreductions in which the carbon and energy source acts as both the electron donor and the electron acceptor. This process is known as fermentation and leads to the formation of several organic end products such as acids and alcohol as well as of gas (carbon dioxide and hydrogen).

Growth and Multiplication of Bacteria:

Bacteria multiply by binary fission (splitting into two). When a bacteria cell reaches a certain size, it divides to form two daughter cells. Nuclear division precedes cell division. The single piece of double stranded DNA reproduces itself exactly. The cell divides by a constrictive or pinching process or by the ingrowth of a transverse septum across the cell. When a bacterial species produces several forms, each with its own characteristic, these variations are called strains.

The growth cycle of bacteria has four major phases, which are as follows:

i. **Lag phase:** during which vigorous metabolic activity occurs but cell don't divide. This can last for a few minutes up to many hours.

ii. **Log phase:** The log phase is when rapid cell division occurs.

iii. **Stationary phase:** It occurs when nutrient depletion or toxic products causes growth to slow.

iv. **Decline or Death phase:** This is the phase when the population decreases due to cell death.[30, 31, 32, 33, 34]

Classification of Bacteria:

Bacteria are mainly classified into phyla (phylum is a scientific classification of organisms).For simplification, bacteria can be grouped into the following:

Bacterial Classification based on shapes:

As already mentioned, before the advent of DNA sequencing, bacteria were classified based on their shapes and biochemical properties. Most of the bacteria belong to three main shapes:

1. Rod shaped bacteria are called bacilli.

2. Sphere shaped bacteria are called cocci.

3. Spiral shaped bacteria are called spirilla.

Bacterial classification based on Aerobic and Anaerobic bacteria:

Bacteria are also classified based on the requirement of oxygen for their survival.

- Bacteria those need oxygen for their survival are called Aerobic bacteria.

- Bacteria those do not require oxygen for survival are called anaerobic bacteria.

- Anaerobic bacteria are found in places like under the surface of earth, deep Ocean.

Bacterial Classification based on Gram Positive and Gram Negative bacteria:

Bacteria are grouped as 'Gram Positive' bacteria and 'Gram Negative' bacteria, which are based on the results of Gram Staining Method in which; an agent is used to bind to the cell wall of the bacteria.

Gram-positive bacteria posses a thick cell wall, containing many layers of peptidoglycan & teichoicacid. Gram-negative bacteria have a relatively thin cell wall consisting of a few layers of peptidoglycan surrounded by a second lipid membrane containing lipo-polysaccharides & lipo-proteins.

Bacterial Classification based on Autotrophic and Heterotrophic Bacteria:

This is one of the most important classification types as it takes into account the most important aspect of bacteria growth and reproduction. They obtain the carbon from carbon-dioxide. Some autotrophs directly use sun-light in order to produce sugar from carbon-dioxide whereas other depend on various chemical reactions. Heterotrophic bacteria obtain carbon and/or sugar from the environment e.g. the living cells or organism.

Classification based on Phyla:

Based on the morphology, DNA sequencing, conditions required and biochemistry, scientists have classified bacteria into phyla:

1) Aquificae: They derived their energy from inorganic molecules & they live in hot Environment 95∘c.

2) Xenobacteria: having ability to survive in high dose of radiation 30,000Gy (1 Gy=100 radiation). A human being can be killed by less than 5Gy.

3) Fibrobacter

4) Bacteroids

5) Firmicutes

6) Planctomycetes: They are unique because they produce stalk. They are budding bacteria.

7) Chrysogenetic

8) Cyanobacteria: photosynthetic organisms found in rock, fresh, salt water.

9) Thermomicrobia

10) Chlorobia: Green sulphur bacteria. They all are obligatory anaerobic phototrophic species.

11) Proteobacteria

12) Spirochaetes: Tightly coiled & slender in shape. They have one or more flagella.

13) Flavobacteria: Found in food processing plants.

14) Fusobacteria: They are filamentous bacteria which secondary colonists on the dental plaque on teeth.

15) Verrucomicrobia

Each phylum further corresponds to number of species and genera of bacteria. The bacteria classification includes bacteria which are found in various types of environments such as sweet water bacteria, ocean water bacteria, bacteria that can survive extreme temperatures (extreme hot as in sulfur water spring bacteria and extreme cold as in bacteria found in Antarctica ice), bacteria that can survive in highly acidic environment, bacteria that can survive highly alkaline environment, aerobic bacteria, anaerobic bacteria, autotrophic bacteria, heterotrophic bacteria, bacteria that can withstand high radiation etc

33.

BACTERIA USED IN EXPERIMENT

1. *Escherichia coli*

Classification:

Kingdom : Bacteria

Phylum   : Proteobacteria

Class   : Gammaproteobacteria

Order   : Enterobacteriales

Family   : Enterobacteriaceae

Genus   : *Escherichia*

Species   : *coli*

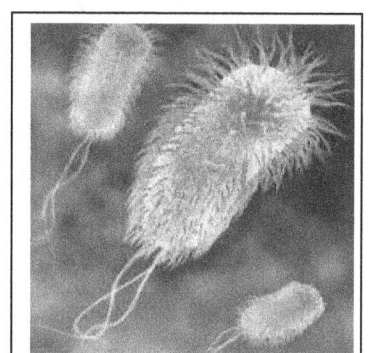

Escherichia coli are facultative anaerobic gram negative rod shaped bacteria that live in the intestinal tracts of animal in health and disease. It are about 1-3× 0.4-0.7 µm in size.

Pathogenesis: *E.coli* are responsible for three types of infections in humans: urinary tract infections (UTI), neonatal meningitis, and intestinal diseases (gastroenteritis), pyogenic infection and septicaemia. The diseases caused (or not caused) by a particular strain of *E.coli* depend on distribution and expression of an array of virulence determinants, including adhesins, invasins, toxins, and abilities to withstand host defences.

2. *Klebsiella pneumoniea*

Classification:

Kingdom : Bacteria
Phylum   : Proteobacteria
Class   : Gammaproteobacteria
Order   : Enterobacteriales
Family   : Enterobacteriaceae
Genus   : *Klebsiella*
Species   : *pneumonia*

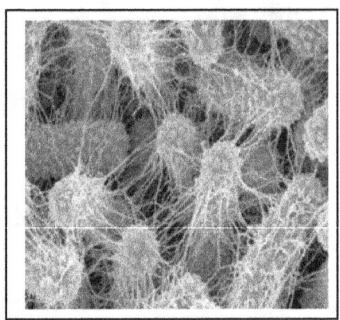

Klebsiella pneumoniea is a gram negative facultative anaerobic non motile bacterium. They are short, plump, straight rods, about 1-2×0.5-0.8 μm in size.

Klebsiella pneumoniea can be found as a commensal in the mouth, upper respiratory tract and intestinal tract of humans and animals. It is also found in moist environment, particularly in hospital. These are also found in plants, water and soil.

Pathogenesis: These organisms are usually opportunistic pathogens that cause nosocomial infection, especially pneumonia and urinary tract infections. It is an important respiratory tract pathogen out side hospital as well.

3. *Proteus vulgaris*

Classification:

Kingdom : Bacteria

Phylum : Proteobacteria

Class   : Gamma Proteobacteria

Order   : Enterobacteriales

Family : Enterobacteriaceae

Genus   : *Proteus*

Species : *vulgaris*

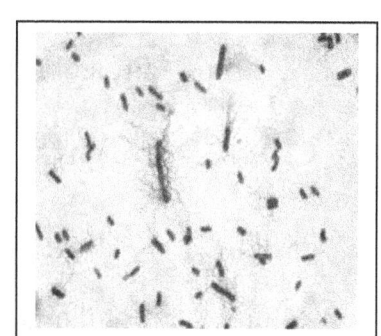

These bacteria are gram negative, rod shaped and motile. These are distinguished from other members of enterobacteriaceae by their ability to produce the enzyme phenylalanins daeminase. The organisms are present in the humans' colon as well as in soil and water.

Pathogenesis: These organisms primarily cause urinary tract infections both community and hospital acquired and wound infections.

4. *Pseudomonas aeruginosa*

Classification:

Kingdom : Bacteria

Phylum   : Proteobacteria

Class   : Gamma Proteobacteria

Order   : Pseudomonadales

Family   : Pseudomonadaceae

Genus   : *Pseudomonas*

Species   : *aeruginosa*

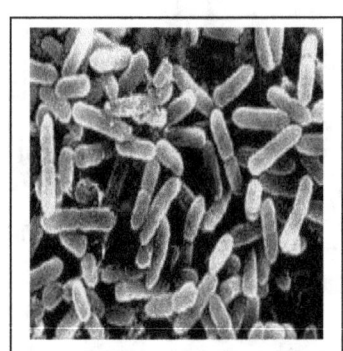

This bacterium is gram negative, aerobic, motile and rod, 1.5-3×0.5 µm in size. It is free living bacterium, commonly found in soil, water and on surface in contact with soil or water, although approximately 10% of people carry it in the normal flora of the colon.

Pathogenesis: It causes urinary tract infections, respiratory system infections, dermatitis, soft tissue infections, bacteremia, bone and join infections, gasterointestinal infections, meningitis and brain abscesses. It is one of the agents responsible for infantile diarrhoea.

5. *Staphylococcus aureus*

Classification:

Kingdom : Bacteria

Phylum : Firmicutes

Class : Bacilli

Order : Bacillales

Family : Staphylococcaceae

Genus : *Staphylococcus*

Species : *aureus*

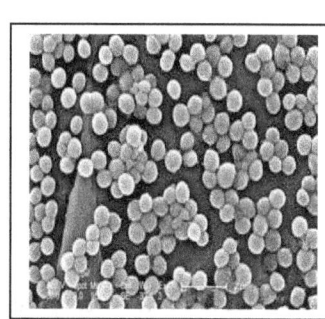

Staphylococci are gram-positive, spherical bacteria, approximately 1µm in diameter that occur in microscopic clusters resembling grapes. Staphylococci are ubiquitous in the human environment and in the normal human flora.

Pathogenesis: Staphylococcus aureus causes a varity of suppurative infections and toxinoses in humans. It causes superficial skin lesions such boils, styes and furunculosis; more serious infections such as pneumonia, mastitis, phlebitis, meningitis, and urinary tract infections; and deep seated infections, such as osteomyelitis and endocarditis. *S.aureus* is a major cause of hospital acquires (nosocomial) infection of surgical wounds. It also causes food poisoning.

6. *Shigella sonnei*

Classification:

Kingdom : Bacteria

Phylum : Proteobacteria

Class   : Gamma proteobacteria

Order   : Enterobacteriales

Family : Enterobacteriaceae

Genus   : *Shigella*

Species : *sonnei*

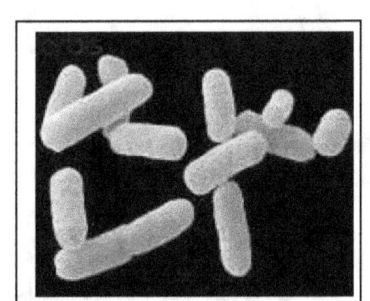

Shigella sonnei is a gram-negative, non-motile, non-spore forming, rod-shaped bacterium, about 0.5×1-3 µm in size, very closely related to *E.coli*.

Pathogenesis: Shigellae are the most effective pathogens among the enteric bacteria. Shigellosis is the only human disease.

7. *Salmonella sp.*

Classification:

Kingdom : Bacteria
Phylum   : Proteobacteria
Class   : Gammaproteobacteria
Order   : Enterobacteriales
Family   : Enterobacteriaceae
Genus   : *Salmonella*
Species : *typhi & paratyphi*

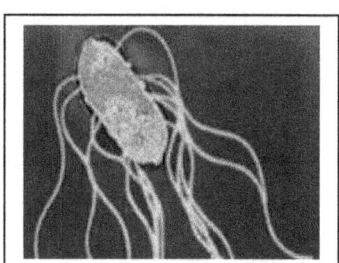
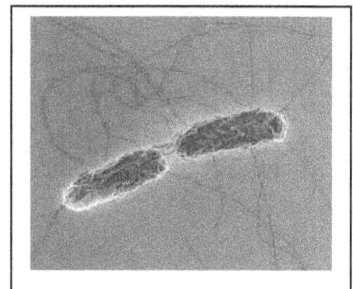

Salmonella typhi

Salmonellae are gram-negative, aerobic, and facultative anaerobic, motile, rod, about 1-3×0.5 μm in size. The principle habitat of salmonellae is the intestinal tract of human and animals.

Pathogenesis: Salmonella species cause entrocolitis or food poisoning, enteric fevers such as typhoid fever (cause by *Salmonella typhi*) and paratyphoid fever(cause by *Salmonella paratyphi*), and septicemia with metastatic abscesses.[30, 32, 34, 35, 36, 37, 38, 39, 40, 41]

Conventional antibiotics and their targets in bacterial cells [42]

At least 17 different classes of antibiotics, synthetic and of microbial origin have been produced up to date.[43] These antibiotics act by a) inhibiting the synthesis of the bacterial cell wall, b) Inhibition of protein synthesis , c) Inhibition of DNA synthesis , d) Inhibition of RNA synthesis , e) Competitive inhibition of folic acid biosynthesis, f) Disorganizing membranes and other mechanisms.[44]

Penicillins and cephalosporins, derived from the fungal species Penicillium chrysogenum and Cephalosporinum *sp.* inhibit the synthesis of the bacterial cell wall by binding to the transpeptidase enzyme thus inhibiting the formation of peptidoglycan. Gram-negative bacteria are in general more resistant than gram-positive bacteria to the actions of antibiotics since they contain an outer membrane with a lipopolysaccharide layer which renders them impermeable to certain antibiotics and bactericidal compounds.[45] Thus the naturally derived penicillin G does not have the ability to penetrate the gram-negative outer membrane. In synthetically modified penicillins (semi-synthetic penicillins) the N-acyl side chain is modified and enables these compounds to penetrate the outer membrane of gram-negative bacteria, and thus semi-synthetic penicillins have a much broader spectrum of activity than penicillin is susceptible to the sections β-lactamases, enzymes produced by penicillin-resistant bacteria. Some semi-synthetic penicillin, such as oxacillin and methicillin, are β-lactamase resistant. The cephalosporins are more resistant than the penicillins to the β-lactamases and thus have a broader spectrum of antibacterial activity [44].The other three main classes of antibiotics. Derived from bacterial source, such as the aminoglycoside and macrolide antibiotics, as well as the tetracyclines inhibit protein synthesis by binding to either the 30S or the 50S subunits of the ribosome.[44]

Purely synthetic antibiotics act as growth analogues, for example the sulfa drugs, which block the synthesis of folic acid, purines, pyurimidins and other compounds. The quinolones act with bacterial DNA gyrase and prevent the gyrase from supercoiling bacterial DNA, which is required for packing DNA in the bacterial cell.[44]

Defence chemicals produced by plants

Higher plants produce a great diversity of chemicals that have antimicrobial activity in vitro.[46] Most of these defence molecules are secondary metabolites, of which at least 12000 have been isolated.[47]There are two broad categories of plant produced antimicrobials. **1) Phytoalexins** are low molecular compounds which are produced in response to microbial, herbivorous or environmental stimuli.[46] These compounds are synthesized de novo, and thus require activation of certain genes and enzymes required for their synthesis.

45

Phytoalexins are chemically diverse and include simple phenylpropanoid derivates, such as flavonoids, isofavonoids, terpenes and polyketides.[48, 49, 50]

2) Phytoanticipins are low molecular compounds which are presents in plants before the challenge by microorganisms or are produced from pre-existing constituents after infection.[46] These phytoanticipin toxins, e.g. phenolic and iridoid glycosides, glucosinolates and saponins are normally stored as less toxic glycosides in the vacuoles of plant cells. If the integrity of the cell is broken when penetrated by the microbe, the glycoside comes into contact with hydrolyzing enzymes present in other compartments of the cell, releasing the toxic aglycone.[51] There is no sharp boundary between phytoalexins and phytoanticipins, and in one plant species a certain chemical can function as a phytoalexin, whereas it has the function of a phytoanticipin in another species. [52,53] The rich diversity of secondary metabolites in plants has partly arisen because of selection for improved defence mechanisms against a broad array of microbes, insects and other plants. Related plants families often make use of similar secondary compounds for defence purposes (isoflavonoids in Leguminosae; sesquiterpenses in Solanaceae). Most antimicrobial secondary metabolites have relatively broad spectrum of activity. The specificity is determined to whether the pathogen has the enzymes necessary to detoxify a particular host product.[46]

DESCRIPTION OF DRUG

RAPHANUS SATIVUS L.

Classification: [54, 55, 56, 57]

Kingdom	:	Plantae
Division	:	Magnoliophyta (angiosperms)
Class	:	Magnoliopsida (dicotyledons)
Order	:	Brassicales
Family	:	Brassicaceae (Cruciferae)
Genus	:	*Raphanus*
Species	:	*sativus*

Vernacular Names: [58, 59, 60, 61 62]

Urdu	:	Mooli
Arabic	:	Bazrul fazl
Persian	:	Tukhm-e-Turb
Hindi	:	Muli
Bengali	:	Mula
Gujarati	:	Mula

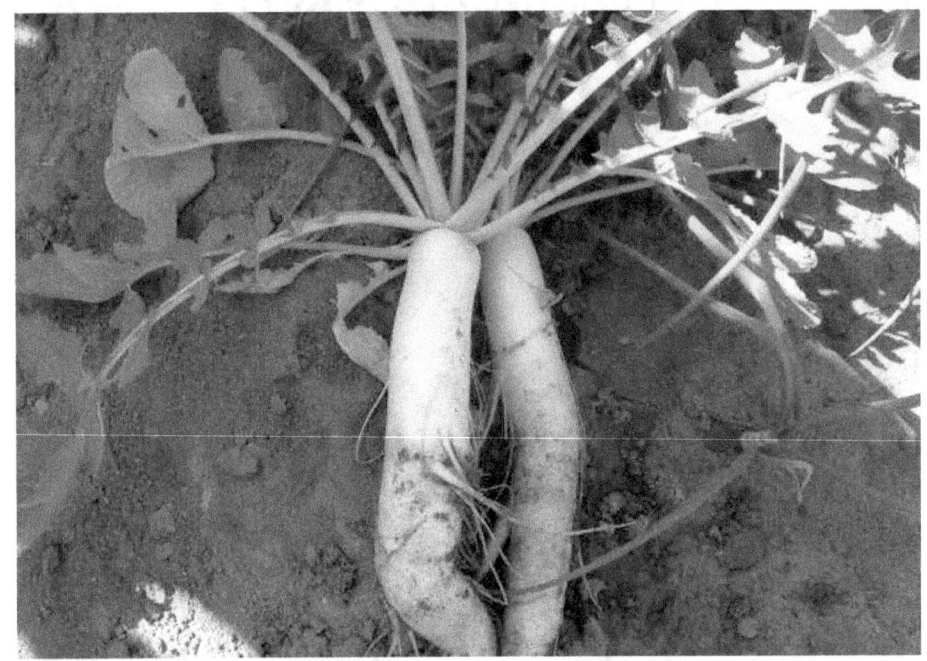

Mooli

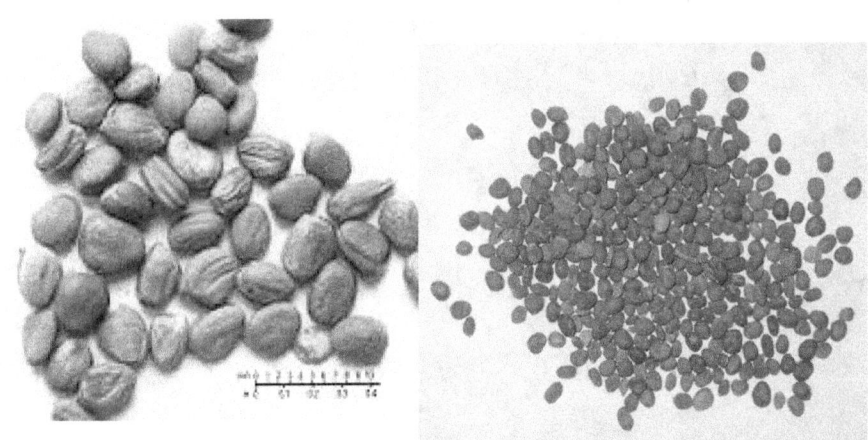

Tukhm-e-Mooli

Kannad	:	Moollangi
Tamil	:	Mullangi
Malayalam	:	Mullank
Marathi	:	Mula
Oriya	:	Mula, rakhyasmula
Punjabi	:	Mulaka, Muli, Mula
Telugu	:	Mullangi
English	:	Radish

Habitat:

Cultivated Beds; While this plant is often grown in vegetable gardens, it is uncommon to find the Garden Radish in the wild. Habitats include dumps, cdgcs of gardens, areas along roadsides and railroads, and waste areas. [60, 61, 63, 72]

Period of Occurrence:

They are in season from October to April and from December to June. [64, 65, 66]

Cultivation and Propagation:

The radish is cultivated in all parts of the country from the coastal plains to the Himalayan ranges up to 3,000 m or even more. In general, the radish is a cool season crop, though there are said to be some indigenous types that can be grown throughout year. There are certain regions in the country, for example, South India, where radish is cultivated all round the year. The main season for sowing in the northern plains for indigenous types is from august to January and for European types from September to March. In the hills they are sown from March to July. The best sowing periods in south India are from April to June in the hills and October to December in the plains.[15, 57, 59, 60, 67, 72]

Parts Used:

Fresh root, leaves, seeds and whole plant.[15, 64, 68, 69]

Morphology:

Radish comes from the Latin *radix,* meaning "root". The descriptive Greek name of the genus *Raphanus* means "quickly appearing" and refers to the rapid germination of these plants.

Radish is an herbaceous plant, of the Brassicaceae family, grown as an annual or biennial, and characterized by a large, fleshy, tuberous tap root and white to purple hermaphrodite flowers clustered in a terminal raceme, cultivated throughout India up to 3,000 m in the Himalayas and other hilly regions.

Stem simple or branched, erect, 20-100cm, basal **leaves** long, lyrately pinnate or pinnatisect, coarsely toothed; cauline leaves simple, linear. **Flowers** in long terminal racemes usually white or lilac with purple veins; **fruits** are a peculiar kind of capsule named siliqua, inflated 25-90 mm long,

50

with a long tapering beak, hardly or irregularly constricted and filled inside with white pith between seeds; **seeds** are oval-shaped, slightly flattened, 2-8, globose, yellow or brown. [15, 57, 59, 60, 63, 64 65, 66, 67 68, 69, 70, 72]

Pharmacognosy of seed:

Macroscopic: Seed reddish brown, irregularly globose, sometimes flattened, 2-4 mm long and 2 mm wide; surface generally smooth and sometimes wrinkled and grooved at micropylar end; taste, oily.

Microscopic: Seed shows testa; consisting of single layer of nearly rectangular cells, covered with thin cuticle, followed by a layer of radially elongated, reddish brown columnar cells, and integument 2-3 layers of compressed, thin-walled, parenchymatous cells; cotyledons and embryo consist of oval to polygonal, thin-walled, parenchymatous cells containing aleurone grains and oil globules.[58]

Temperament: [78, 79, 80, 81, 82 83, 84, 85, 86]

Hot 3°, Dry 2°

Taste: [78, 79, 80, 81, 82 83, 84, 85, 86]

It tastes Hot, Sharp, Bitter and Irritative.

Odour: [78, 79, 80, 81, 82 83, 84, 85, 86]

Pungent

Actions: 15, 16, 17, 57, 59, 60, 61, 63, 64, 65, 66, 68, 69, 70, 72, 73, 78, 79, 80, 81, 82 83, 84, 85, 86

- Carminative

- Diuretic

- Stomachic

- Laxative

- Purgative

- Expectorant

- Peptic

- Emmenagogues

- Cholagogue

- Antitussive

- Anthelmintic

- Antibacterial

- Antifungal

- Antiscorbutic

- Antispasmodic

- Astringent

- Emetic

Therapeutic uses: 15, 16, 17, 57, 59, 60, 61, 63, 64, 65, 66, 68, 69, 70, 72, 73, 78, 79, 80, 81, 82 83, 84, 85, 86

- Piles

- Gastrodynic pain

- Inflammations

- Cardiac Disorders

- Amenorrhoea

- Hiccough

- Spleen Paralysis

- Oedema

- Dysentery

- Diarrhoea

- Asthma

- Freckles

- Lumbago

- Oliguria

- Eruptive Fevers

- Tympanites of Abdomen

- Malnutrition

- Cough

- Cholera

- Flatulence

- Acidity

- Ringworm

- Skin eruptions

- Prolapse of Rectum

- Earache

- Leprosy

• Syphlitic diseases

• Tumours

• Gall Bladder diseases

• Liver disorders

Pharmacological Activity: [15, 16, 17, 57, 59, 60, 61, 63, 64, 65, 66, 68, 69, 70, 72, 73, 78, 79, 80, 81, 82, 83, 84, 85, 86]

• The juice of the fresh leaves is used as a diuretic and laxative.

• The roots stimulate the appetite and digestion, having a tonic and laxative effect upon the intestines and indirectly stimulating the flow of bile.

• Consuming radish generally results in improved digestion, but some people are sensitive to its acridity and robust action.

• The leaves, seeds and old roots are used in the treatment of asthma and other chest complaints.

• It is taken internally in the treatment of indigestion, abdominal bloating, wind, acid regurgitation, diarrhoea and bronchitis.

• It is crushed and used as a poultice for burns, bruises and smelly feet.

• It is an excellent food remedy for stone, gravel and scorbutic conditions.

•Seed of radish contain bleaching substances; therefore, the emulsion with water is applied to over face to remove the blackheads and freckles.

•It is applied to cure ringworm.

•A teaspoonful of the seeds boiled in cow's milk is given every night as a medicine to cure impotency, immature ejaculation etc.

•Decoction of seeds is given as a safe emetic in children suffering from whooping cough.

•Cardio protective investigation of its fruit powder has performed in rabbit.[74]

•Hepatoprotective activity has performed in wistar albino rat.[75]

•Gastroprotective effect of radish on experimental gastric ulcer models in rat has done.[76]

•Antiurolithiatic activity of radish aqueous extract on rat has done.[77]

Muzir (Adverse effect): [78, 79, 80, 81, 82 83, 84, 85, 86]

• It may produces nausea, unease.

•It may produce flatulence, headache and harm to individuals with cold temperament.

•Excessive use of seeds is regarded as harmful for kidneys and liver and for warm temperament individuals.

Musleh (Corrective): [17,78, 79, 80, 81, 82 83, 84, 85, 86]

Caraway (*Carum carvi* L.), Common salt and Honey for seed

Badal (Substitutes): [78, 79, 80, 81, 82 83, 84, 85, 86]

Tukhm-e-Sarsoo (seed of Mustard)

Compound Preparations: [91, 92, 93, 94]

- Sufoof hajr-ul-yhud

- Roghan Turb

- Laboob Kabeer

- Arq Hazim

- Majoon Piyaz

- Majoon Murawwihul Arwah

Phytochemials present in Mooli (*Raphanus sativus* L.)

• **4-METHYLSULFOXIDEBUTEN-(3)-YL-CYANIDE** *Seed* 200 ppm;

• **ALANINE** *Root* 220 - 4,265 ppm

• **ARGININE** *Plant*:

• **ASCORBIC-ACID** *Fruit* 690 - 7,822 ppm *Leaf* 810 - 7,043 ppm *Root* 226 - 6,216 ppm

• **ASPARTIC-ACID** *Root* 480 - 9,300 ppm

• **BETA-CAROTENE** *Fruit* 0.3 - 26.2 ppm *Leaf* 24.7 - 214 ppm *Root* 1 ppm;

• **BETA-HEXYLALDEHYDE** *Seed*:

• **CAFFEIC-ACID** *Root* 91 ppm;

• **CARBOHYDRATES** *Fruit* 54,000 - 701,000 ppm *Leaf* 57,000 - 496,000 ppm *Root* 36,000 - 757,000 ppm

• **CYSTINE** *Root* 50 - 970 ppm

• **DIALLYL-SULFIDE** *Root*:

• **ERUCIC-ACID** *Seed*:

• **FAT** *Fruit* 3,000 - 50,000 ppm *Leaf* 6,000 - 52,000 ppm *Root* 1,000 - 187,000 ppm *Seed* 298,000 - 410,000 ppm

• **FERULIC-ACID** *Root 16 ppm*

• **FIBER** *Fruit 11,000 - 147,000 ppm* **Leaf** *11,000 - 96,000 ppm* **Root** *5,200 - 176,000 ppm*

• **FOLACIN** *Root 0.3 - 5.8 ppm*

• **GLUCOBRASSICIN** *Plant*:

• **GLUCOCAPPARIN** *Seed*:

• **GLUCOLEPIDIIN** *Seed*:

• **GLUCOPUTRANJIVIN** *Root*:

• **GLUCORAPHANIN** *Root*:

• **GLUTAMIC-ACID** *Root 1,320 - 25,580 ppm*

• **GLYCEROL-SINAPATE** *Seed*:

• **GLYCINE** *Root 220 - 4,265 ppm*

• **HISTIDINE** *Root 130 - 2,520 ppm*

• **INDOLE-ACETIC-ACID** *Root*:

• **INDOLEACETONITRILE** *Root*:

• **ISOBUTYRALDEHYDE** *Leaf*:

- **ISOLEUCINE** *Root* 300 - 5,815 ppm

- **L-SULFORAPHENE** *Root*:

- **LEUCINE** *Root* 370 - 7,170 ppm

- **LINOLEIC-ACID** *Root* 160 - 3,100 ppm

- **LINOLENIC-ACID** *Root* 290 - 5,620 ppm

- **LYSINE** *Root* 350 - 6,785 ppm

- **METHIONINE** *Root* 70 - 1,355 ppm

- **METHYL-MERCAPTAN** *Seed*:

- **MYRISTIC-ACID** *Root*:

- **N-BUTYRALDEHYDE** *Leaf*:

- **NIACIN** *Fruit* 2 - 59 ppm *Leaf* 40 - 348 ppm *Root* 3 - 68 ppm

- **OLEIC-ACID** *Root* 160 - 3,100 ppm

- **OXALIC-ACID** *Root* 92 ppm;

- **P-COUMARIC-ACID** *Root* 91 ppm;

- **PALMITIC-ACID** *Root* 260 - 5,040 ppm

- **PANTOTHENIC-ACID** *Root* 0.8 - 18 ppm

•**PHENYLALANINE** *Root 230 - 4,455 ppm*

•**PHYTOSTEROLS** *Root 70 - 1,355 ppm*

•**PROLINE** *Root 180 - 3,490 ppm*

•**PROTEIN** *Fruit 13,000 - 257,000 ppm Leaf 33,000 - 287,000 ppm Root 5,260 - 182,000 ppm Seed 236,000 - 336,000 ppm*

•**PUTRESCINE** *Leaf*:

•**RAPHANIN** *Seed*:

•**RAPHANUSIN-A** ,B, C,D *Root*:

•**RIBOFLAVIN** *Fruit 0.3 - 5.3 ppm Leaf 2.6 - 24 ppm Root 0.3 - 9.3 ppm*

•**S-METHYL-L-CYSTEINSULFOXIDE** *Root*:

•**SERINE** *Root 210 - 4,070 ppm*

•**SINAPIC-ACID** *Root*:

•**SINIGRIN** *Seed*:

•**SPERMINE** *Leaf*:

•**SPERMINIDINE** *Leaf*:

•**STEARIC-ACID** *Root 40 - 775 ppm*

- **THREONINE** *Root* *290 - 5,620 ppm*

- **TRIACONTANE** *Seed*:

- **TRYPTOPHAN** *Root* *40 - 775 ppm*

- **TYROSINE** *Root* *130 - 2,520 ppm*

- **VALINE** *Root* *320 - 6,200 ppm*

- **VIT-B-6** *Root* *0.7 - 14.5 ppm*

- Traces elements (Aluminium, Barium, lithium, Manganese, Silicon, Titanium and Iodine) [18, 60, 87, 88, 89, 90, 111]

STANDARDIZATION OF TUKHM-E MOOLI[58, 95, 96, 97]

Powder: Brownish-yellow; show fragments of testa with hexagonal, thin-walled epidermal cells in surface view; oval to polygonal, thin-walled, parenchymatous cells of embryo, no oil globules and aleurone grains are present.

Moisture content	0.486%
Total Ash value	3.54-3.67 gm %
Acid insoluble Ash	0.29 gm %
Alcohol soluble extractive	8.55 - 9.27 gm %
Water soluble extractive	10.13 - 12.65 gm %
P^H Value 1%	5.88 - 5.90
10%	5.87 - 5.88
Bacterial load	2×10^2
Fungal load	1×10^2
Bulk Density	0.76
Heavy Metal	Nil
Aflatoxin	Nil
Chemical Constituents	Fixed oil and Volatile oil[58, 95, 96,]

Fluorescence Study:

Extract	UV 254 nm	UV 366 nm	Visible Region
Pet. ether	Pale Yellow	Pale Yellow	Yellow
Chloroform	Pale Yellow	Pale Yellow	Pale Yellow
Ethyl Acetate	Pale Yellow	Light Blue	Pale Yellow
Ethanol	Pale Yellow	Light Blue	Pale Yellow

Methanol	Pale Yellow	Light Blue	Pale Yellow
Dist. Water	Blue	Yellow Green	Dull White

Powder Study of the drug:

Extract	UV 254 nm	UV 366nm	Visible Region
Powder as such	Green Yellow	Pale Yellow	Yellow
Conc.H$_2$SO$_4$	Black	Black	Reddish Brown
Conc. HCL	Black	Dark Green	Off White
NaOH in MeOH	Dark Green	Pale Yellow	Yellow
Conc. HNO$_3$	Black	Black	Yellow
Glacial Acetic Acid	Black	Light Blue	Off White

Screening test for Secondary Metabolites in solvent extract of

Raphanus sativus L. Seed: [95, 96, 97]

Secondary Metabolites	Name of Test	Results (+/-)							
Alkaloids	Dragendroff's								
Flavonoids	Shinoda NaOH								
Glycosides	Conc.H_2SO_4 Aq NaOH								
Carbohydrates	Benedict's Molisch's								
Phenol	Ferric chloride Aq. lead acetate								
Saponins	Foam								
Sterols	Salkowski								
Tannins	Ferric chloride								
Proteins	Millon's								

66

Et= Ethanol, **Mt**= Methanol, **Ea**= Ethyl acetate, **Ch**= Chloroform, **Ben**= Benzene, **Aq**=Aqueous, **H**=Hot, **C**=Cold

TLC

TLC of the alcoholic extract on silica gel 'G' plate using Toluene: Ethyl acetate (9:1) shows under U.V. (366 nm) a fluorescent zone at Rf. 0.95 (blue). On exposure to Iodine vapour five spots appear at Rf. 0.17, 0.31, 0.39, 0.70, and 0.95 (all yellow). On spraying with vanillin-sulphuric acid reagent and healing the plate at 105°C for ten minutes four spots appears at Rf. 0.17, 0.31, 0.39, and 0.95 (all violet). [110]

HPTLC Analytical analysis of *Raphanus sativus* L:

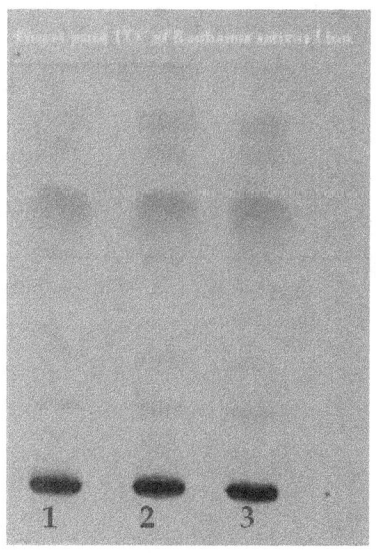

At Visible range

Figure 1: TLC chromatogram of *Raphaus sativus* at visible range.

HPTLC Profile:

Methanolic drug extract spotted on silica gel "G" plate and developed the plate using Toluene: Ethyl Acetate: Methanol (7: 2: 1) mobile phase shows 11 spots under visible region at 350 nm with Rf values 0.09, 0.19, 0.25, 0.37, 0.56, 0.58, 0.68, 0.70, 0.80, 0.85 and 0.97 (all brown colour spots)

Table 1: Peak list of *Raphanus sativus* L. densitogram at visible region at 350nm with Rf. values of the spots.

Peak no	Y-Pos	Area	Area (%)	Height	Rf values
1	8.7	1048.41	35.2	377.42	0.09
2	12.8	37.82	1.3	50.49	0.19
3	15.7	35.65	1.2	50.76	0.25
4	20.6	137.24	4.6	86.93	0.37
5	28.6	71.51	2.4	66.05	0.56
6	29.5	36.46	1.2	74.39	0.58
7	33.6	728.85	24.5	263.48	0.68
8	34.2	253.96	8.5	259.08	0.70
9	38.6	239.52	8.0	130.17	0.80
10	40.9	154.60	5.2	147.78	0.85
11	45.7	232.03	7.8	206.74	0.97

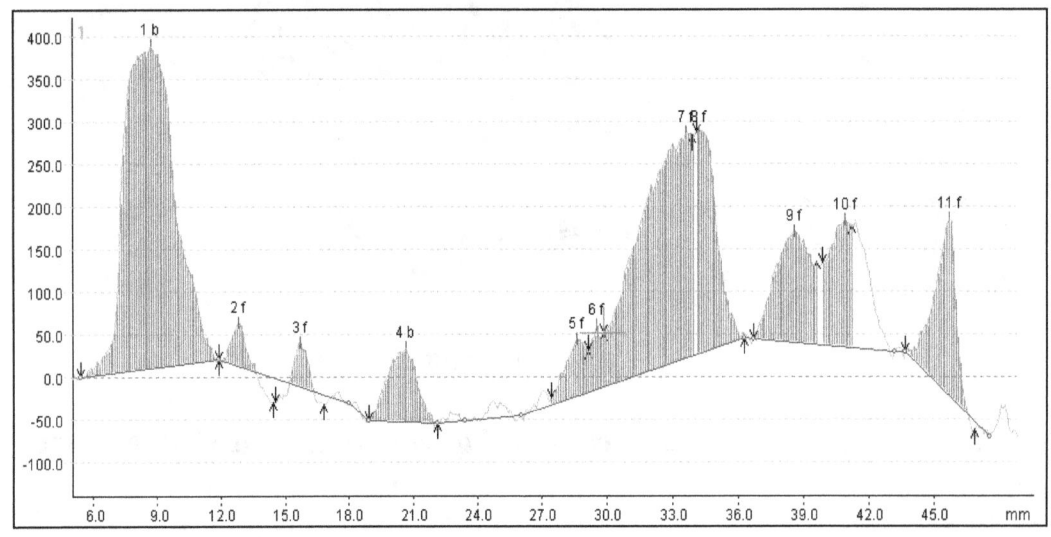

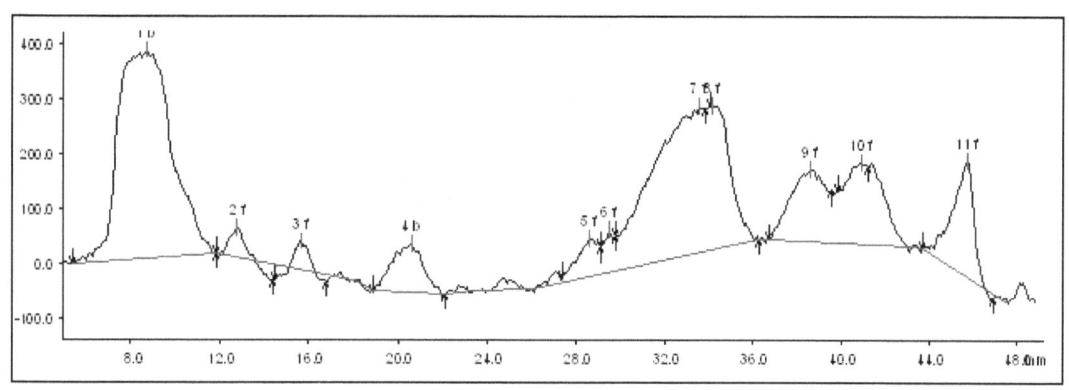

HPTLC Analytical analysis of *Raphanus* HHPTLC Analytical analysis of *Raphanus sativus* L:

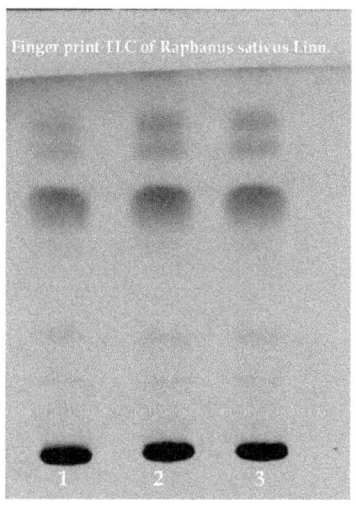

At UV 254nm

Figure 1: TLC chromatogram of *Raphaus sativus* at UV 254nm.

HPTLC Profile:

Methanolic drug extract spotted on silica gel "G" plate and developed the plate using Toluene: Ethyl Acetate: Methanol (7: 2: 1) mobile phase shows seven spots under UV at 254 nm with Rf values at 0.02, 0.21, 0.33, 0.68, 0.87, 0.90 and 0.98 (all black)

Table 1: Peak list of *Raphanus sativus* L. densitogram at UV at 254 nm with Rf. values of the spots.

Peak no	Y-Pos	Area	Area (%)	Height	Rf values
1	6.6	2764.72	38.0	1477.30	0.02
2	13.9	76.92	1.1	92.72	0.21
3	18.4	69.70	1.0	60.43	0.33
4	32.0	1347.29	18.5	368.13	0.68
5	39.2	1172.66	16.1	397.19	0.87
6	40.2	264.77	3.6	401.31	0.90
7	43.4	1584.11	21.8	701.76	0.98

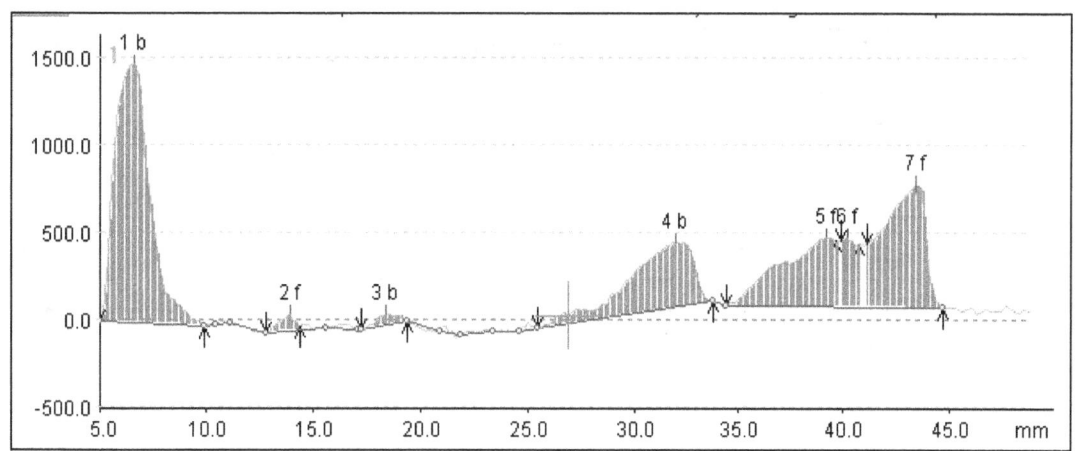

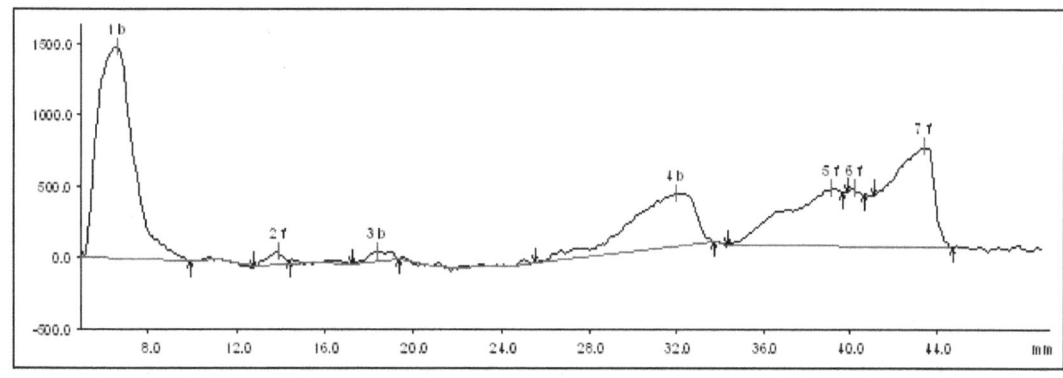

DESAGA ProQuant: Densitogram + Peaklist

Chromatogram:	Measurement - Raphinus seeds meoh ext tol ea meoh 721 254nm	ID-Number:	04802-1309841307-1
Created by:	Rasheed NMA, DSRU	Date/Time:	07/05/2011 10:18:27 AM
Comment:			

Method:	Raphinus seeds meoh ext tol ea meoh 721 254nm	ID-Number:	04802-1309841307-1
Created by:	Rasheed NMA, DSRU	Date/Time:	07/05/2011 10:18:06 AM

Lane 1: Type: Standard 1   Name: Raphinus   X-Position: 5.0 mm

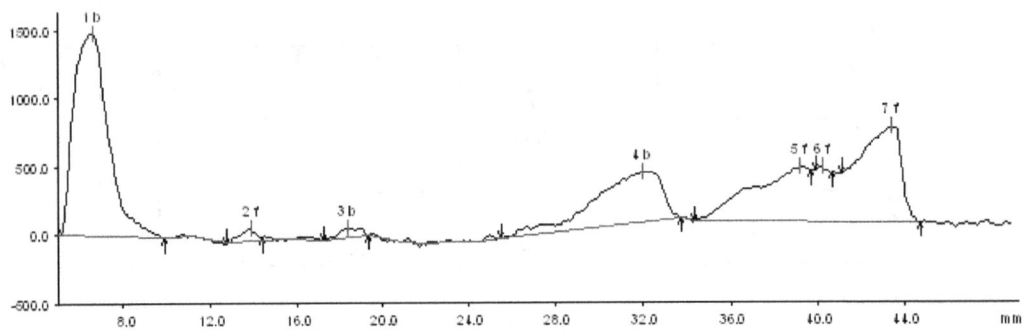

Lane: 1	Type: Standard 1	Name: Raphinus			X-Position: 5.0 mm		
Peak	Component name	y-Pos [mm]	Area	Area[%]	Height	Type	Rf
1	:	6.6	2764.72	38.0	1477.30	b	0.02
2	:	13.9	76.92	1.1	92.72	f	0.21
3	:	18.4	69.70	1.0	60.43	b	0.33
4	:	32.0	1347.29	18.5	368.13	b	0.68
5	:	39.2	1172.66	16.1	397.19	f	0.87
6	:	40.2	264.77	3.6	401.31	f	0.90
7	:	43.4	1584.11	21.8	701.76	f	0.98

72

PART - II

AIMS & OBJECTIVE

• Different parts of the plants have been widely used since ancient times to prevent or cure infectious diseases. Several studies on plants have revealed the presence of antibacterial compounds. The susceptibility and resistance towards a particular antibacterial compound differ from one strain to another strain, so new plants should have to be tested to assess the antibacterial activity against pathogens to carry out to test the antibacterial activity of Tukhm-e-Mooli (seed of *Raphanus sativus* L.).

• To develop a safe and cost effective antibacterial agent.

• To assess the antibacterial property.

• To prove the efficacy of Unani drug Tukhm-e-Mooli on modern scientific parameter.

MATERIALS AND METHODS

Plant Materials:

The samples of seeds of *Raphanus sativus* (Tukhm-e-Mooli) were collected from market and were properly identified authenticated on the basis of literary description available in the Unani classic as well as modern literature by Hk. Mohd Yadullah renowned Unani practitioner and Dr. V.C. Gupta, Deputy Director (Botany) CRIUM, Hyderabad.

Preparation of plant extract:

Different extracts of *Raphanus sativus* seeds were prepared for analysis in the presentstudy.(a)Ethanol(b)Methanol(c)EthylAcetate(d)Chloroform(e)benzene (f)Aqueous Hot (g)Aqueous Cold.

10gms powdered drug soaked in 100 ml of different solvents for 24 hrs & filtered through whattmans filter paper No.1. The filtrate was concentrated by evaporation of solvent on hot plate and water bath at room temperature. All extracts were stored at 4^0C until further use.

Preparation of Test Sample:

A stock solution of the extracts was prepared at the concentration of 100mg/ml and store at 2^0C till further use.

Source and Maintenance of Organisms:

A total 8 strains including gram positive and gram negative bacteria were selected to assess the susceptibility test against the drug extract. The strains were obtained from Institute of Microbial Technology (IMTECH), Chandigarh, India. They were sub cultured on nutrient agar for every 15 days and maintained on nutrient agar slants at 4^0C. Fresh inoculums were taken for the test.

TABLE - BACTERIAL STRAIN USED IN EXPERIMENTS

S.No.	BACTERIA	STRAIN	TYPE
1.	*Escherichia coli*	Gram negative	ATCC 25922
2.	*Klebsiella pneumoniae*	Gram negative	ATCC 27736
3.	*Proteus vulgaris*	Gram negative	ATCC 6380
4.	*Pseudomonas aeruginosa*	Gram negative	ATCC 27853
5.	*Staphylococcus aureus*	Gram positive	ATCC 25923
6.	*Shigella sonnei*	Gram negative	ATCC 25931
7.	*Salmonella paratyphi*	Gram negative	ATCC 9150
8.	*Salmonella typhi*	Gram negative	ATCC 25241

Medias used in experiment:

Medium: it is defined as any substance or material that will enable microorganisms to grow & multiply. A common nutrient medium used for cultivation of bacteria consist of beef extract & peptone in water and is called a liquid medium or broth. All media (broth) provided C, N, Mineral and other growth factors for the growth of microorganism. The liquid medium can b made into solid medium by adding agar-agar (15 to 20%) which acts as a solidifying agent. This substance commonly called agar. Agar is a complex carbohydrate derived from algae of genus gelidium.

1 .Nutrient broth: Himedia

M002-5009

13.0gm of nutrient broth dissolved in 1000ml of distilled water. Dispense as desired, Sterilized by autoclaving at 15lbs pressure (121°C) for required time.

2. Muellar Hinton Agar: Himedia

M173-500gm

This medium was originally formulated for the isolation of pathogenic species. Now days it is more commonly used in microbial assay.

Beef infusion form	300ml
Casein acid hydrolysate	17.5gm
Starch	1.5gms

Agar	10gm
Distilled water	1liter

The bacterial culture were grown in Nutrient Broth and incubated at 37^0C for 24hours, followed by frequent sub culturing on fresh media and were used as test bacteria. Each organism was freshly cultured prior to susceptibility testing by transferring them in to a separate Petri dish containing Muellar Hinton Nutrient Agar incubated over night at 37^0C.

Evaluation of Antibacterial Activity by Agar Well Diffusion:

Antibacterial activities of the extracts were determined by agar well diffusion method. [98, 99 100]

Aim:

To evaluate the plant secondary metabolites sensitivity of Bacterial strains by agar well diffusion method.

Material required:

Bacterial cultures, Drug extracts of Different solvents, Petri plates, Borer, Micropipettes, standard antibiotics (Chloramphenicol and Ciprofloxacin)

Procedure:

Muellar Hinton agar was prepared from a commercially available dehydrated base according to Manufactures instruction. After autoclaving allow it to cool for 5,10mins. After that pour the freshly prepared media in to Petri plates (more than half) the agar medium should be allow cooling at room temperature & stored the plates in refrigerator at 4°C until further use.

Preparation of Inoculums:

•Select & label test cultures that are to be used for (plant extract) Sensitivity Assay.

•Prepare nutrient agar plates.

•3-4 colonies should be selected from the agar plate culture.

•The top of the each colony is touched with loop & transferred in to a test tube containing4-5 ml nutrient broth.

•The test tubes which containing broth cultured are incubated at 37°C until it achieves the turbidity.

Inoculation of test plate:

All strains were first grown in Mueller Hinton broth (MHB) under shaking condition for 4 h 37°C and after the incubation period 0.1ml of the test inoculum was spread evenly with a sterile glass spreader on Mueller Hinton Agar (MHA) plates. The seeded plates were allowed to dry in the incubator at 37°C.

Creating wells and pouring extracts:

Wells were made using sterile 6 mm cork borer in the inoculated MHA plates. The wells were filled with 200µl of the extracts (re-suspended in respective

Solvents) and negative controls 1:1 (solvent: water). The concentration of stock

Extracts was 100 mg /ml. The inoculated plates were incubated at 37^0C for 24 hrs.

Reading plates and results:

The plates were observed for the presence of inhibition of bacterial growth that was indicated by a clear zone around the well. The size of zone of inhibition was measured and the bacterial activity was expressed in term of average diameter of the zone of inhibition in millimetres. The results were compared with the standard antibiotics, Chloramphenicol (25mcg) and Ciprofloxacin (25mcg). The photographs were taken in U.V-visible documentation system.

Different categories for microbial assay testing:

Susceptible:

The "susceptible" category implies that isolates are inhibited by the usually achievable concentrations of antimicrobial agent when the recommended dosage is used for the site of infection.

More than 12mm -highly sensitive

Intermediate:

'The "intermediate" category includes isolates with antimicrobial MICs that approach usually attainable blood and tissue levels and for which response rates may be lower than for susceptible isolates. The intermediate category implies clinical efficacy in body sites where the drugs are physiologically concentrated (e.g. in urine) or when a higher than normal dosage of a drug can be used. This category also includes a buffer zone, which should prevent small, uncontrolled, technical factors from causing major discrepancies in interpretations, especially for drugs with narrow pharamacotoxicity margins.

6-12mm - Intermediate.

Resistant:

'The "resistant" category implies that isolates are not inhibited by the usually achievable concentrations of the agent with normal dosage schedule.

Less than 6mm - Resistant

OBSERVATION AND RESULTS

The present study "Antibacterial activity of Tukhm-e-Mooli" has carried out on eight different gram-negative (*E.coli, K.pneumoniea, P.valgaris, Ps.aeruginosa, S.sonnie, S.paratyphi, S.typhi*) and gram-positive (*Staphylococcus aureus*) bacterial strains.

Results obtained in the present study revealed that tested medicinal plant extracts posses potential antibacterial activity against all selected bacteria (agar well diffusion method). Among all the extracts Ethanolic and Methanolic extracts showed maximum antibacterial activity against all the bacterial strain used with a zone of inhibition ranging from 12-21mm and the least activity was observed in Aqueous cold extract with zone of inhibition ranges from 7-9mm.The test results were compared with standard antibiotics Chloramphenicol and Ciprofloxacin.

Statistical Analysis: The calculations of antibacterial activity were determined by Standard Deviation (SD) and mean of replicates.

Result: Graphical representation

(1)

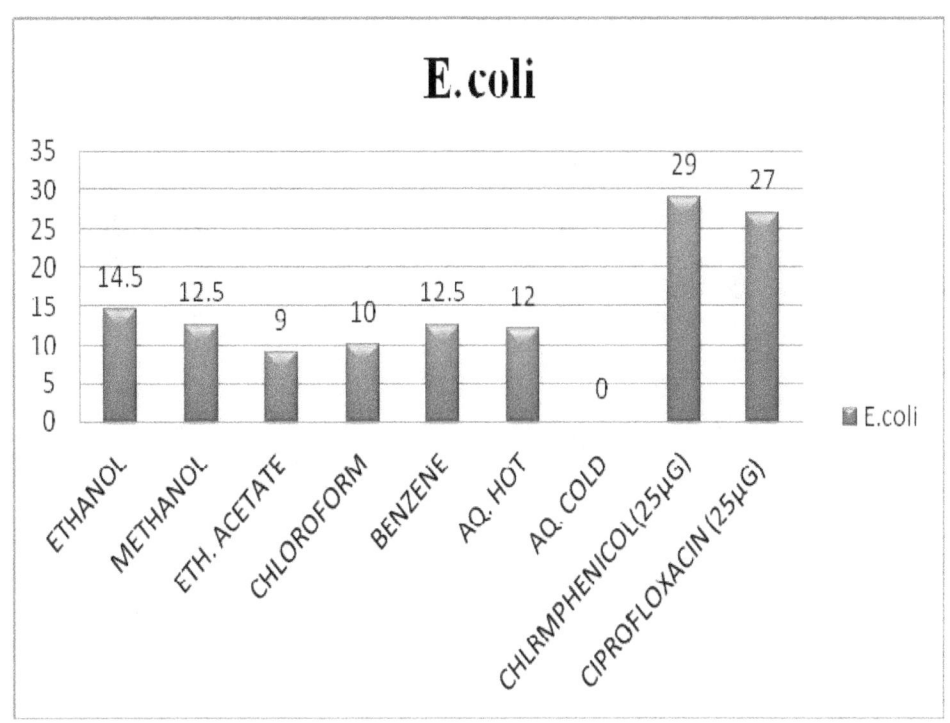

(2)

(3)

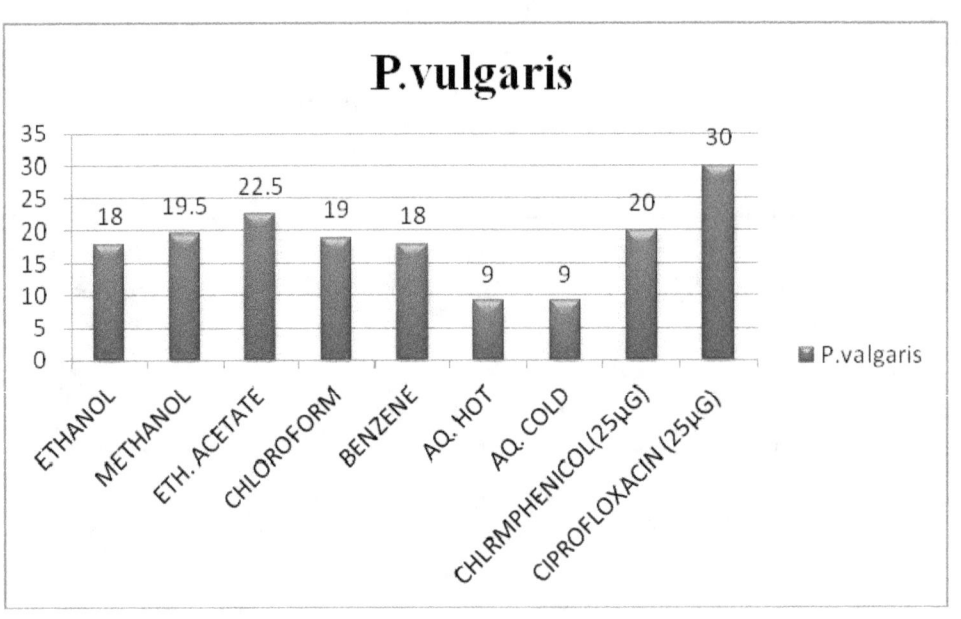

(4)

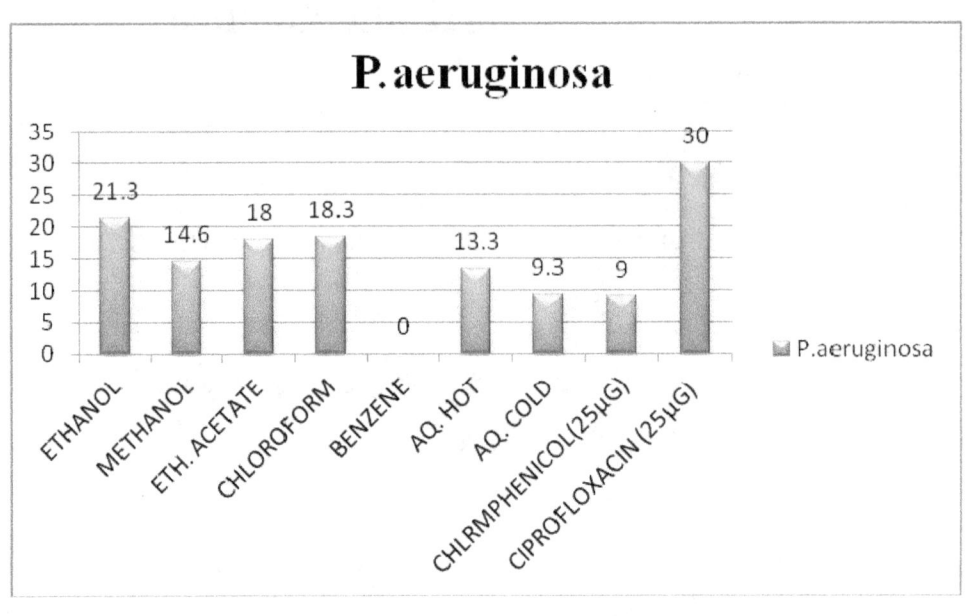

(5)

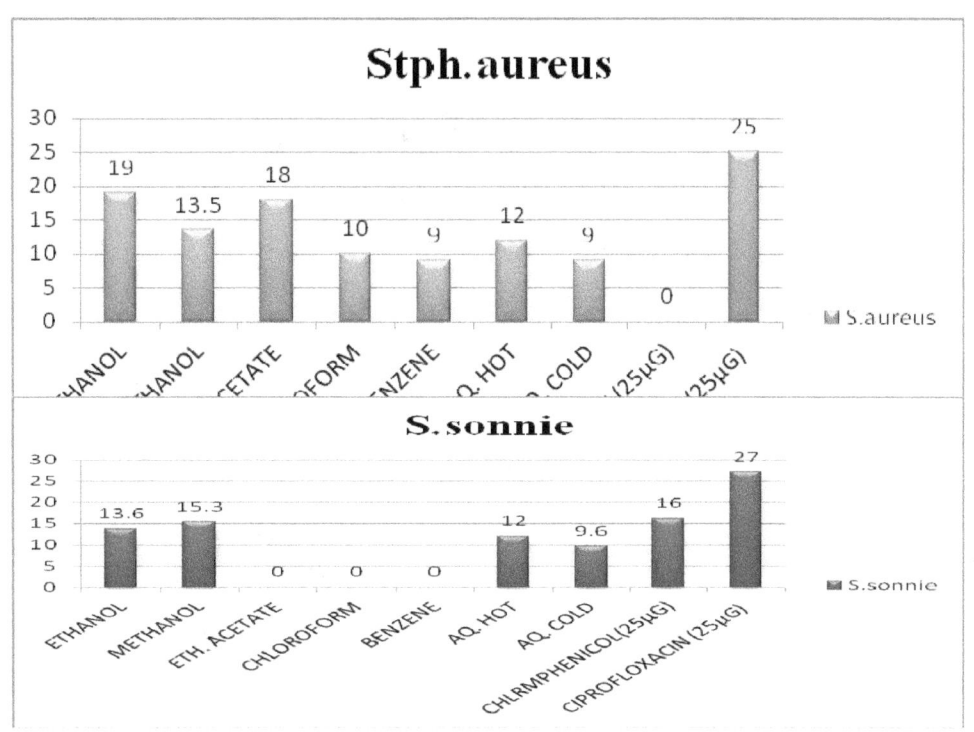

(6)

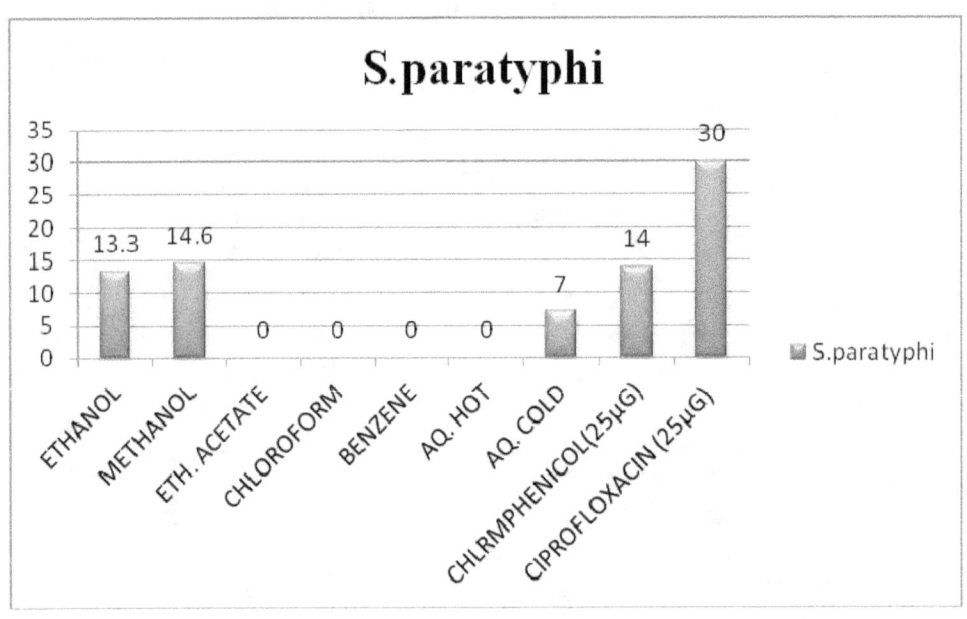

(7)

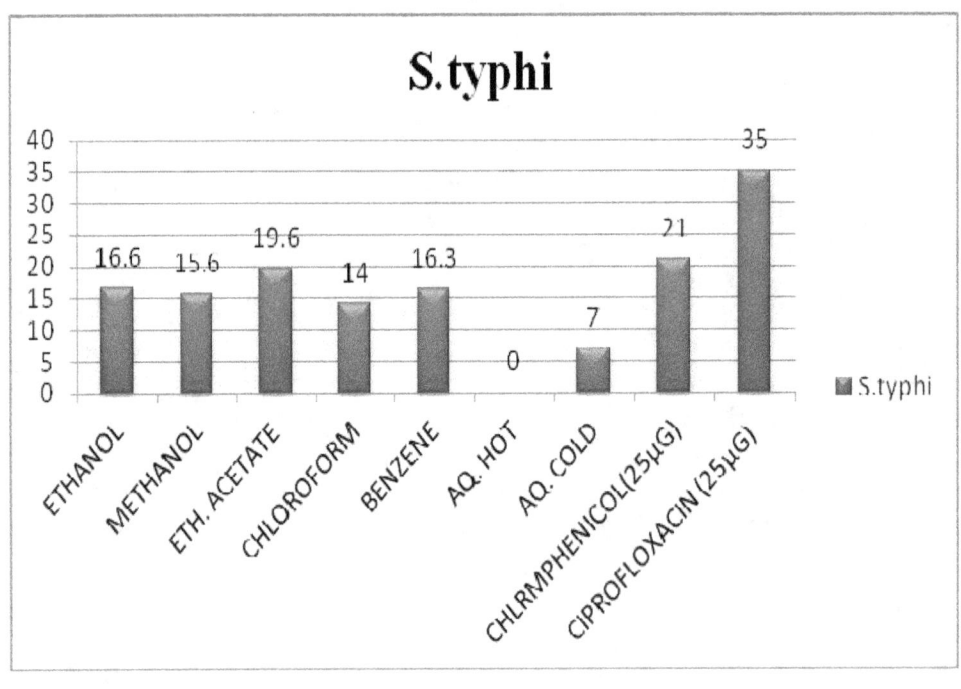

Anti Bacterial activity:

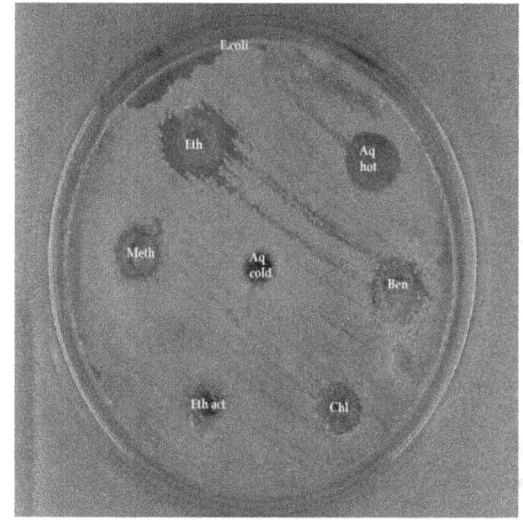

E.coli

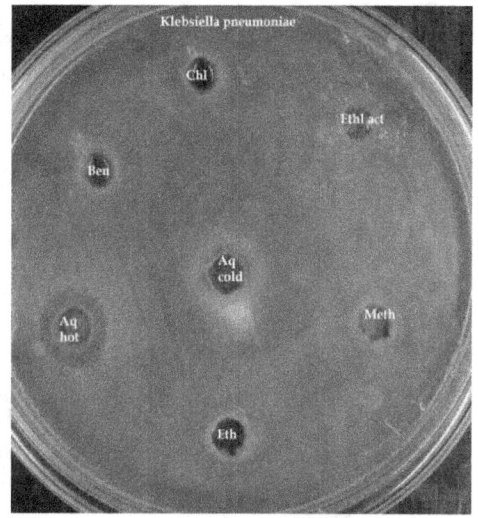

Klebsiella pneumonie

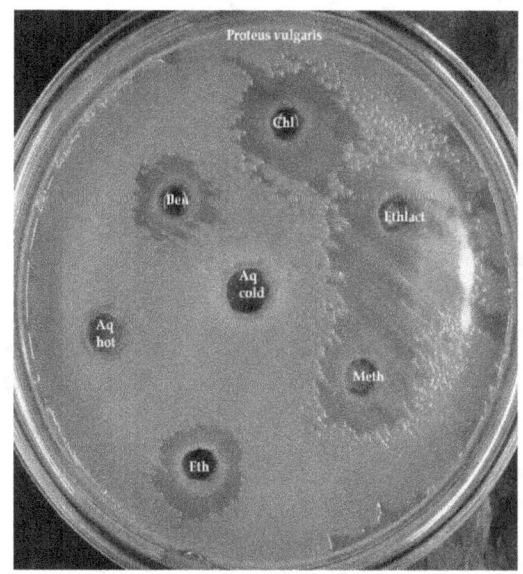

Proteus vulgaris

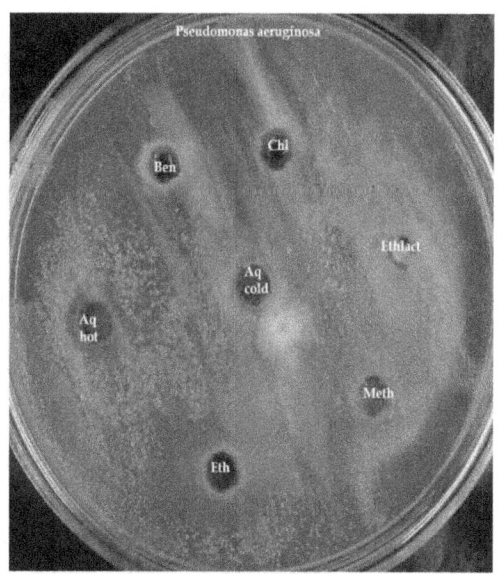

Pseudomonas aeruginosa

Anti Bacterial activity:

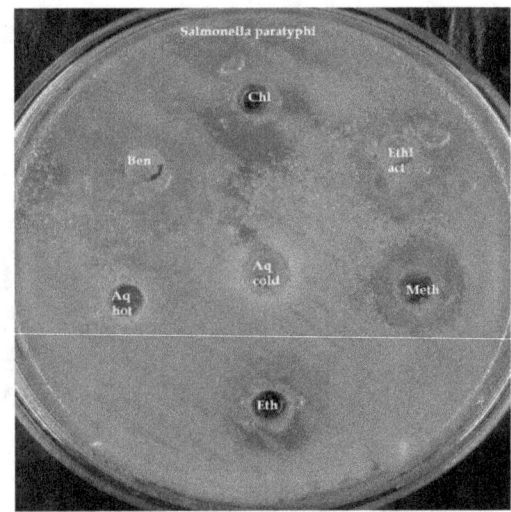

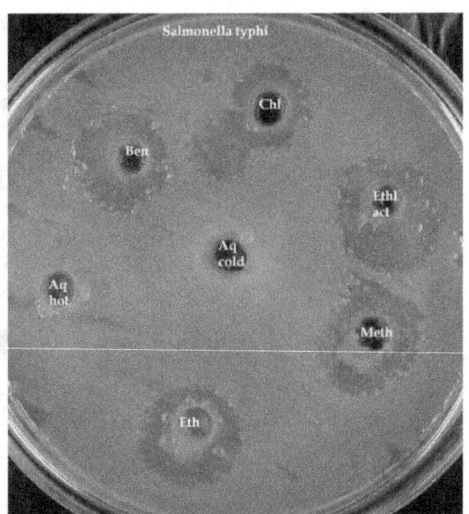

Salmonella paratyphi   *Salmonella typhi*

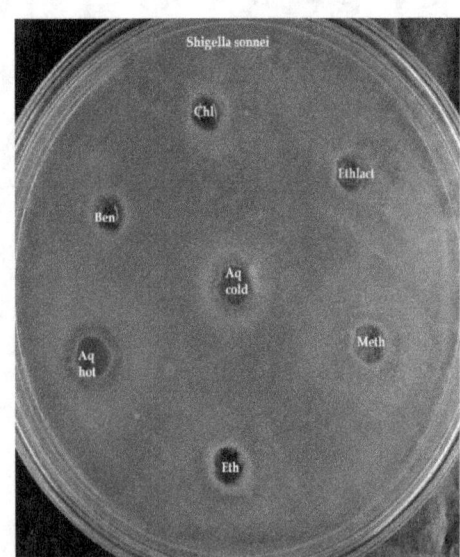

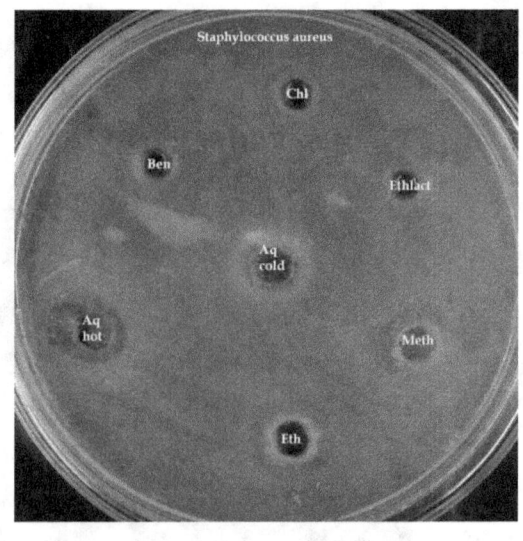

Shigella sonnei   *Staphylococcus aureus*

Positive Control:

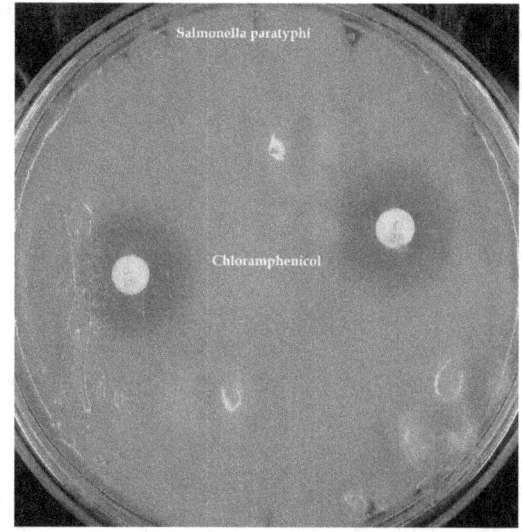

Salmonella paratyphi

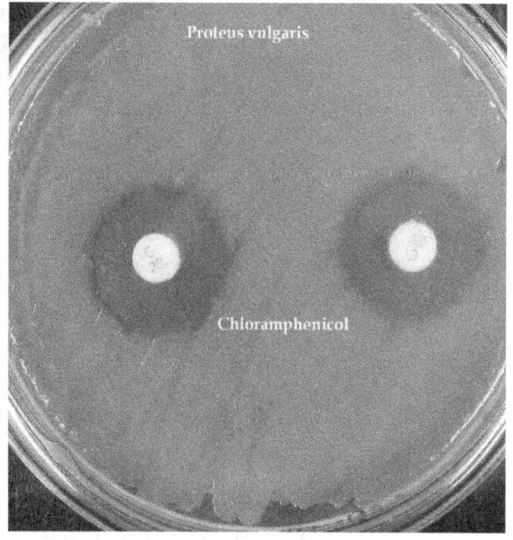

Pseudomonas aeruginosa

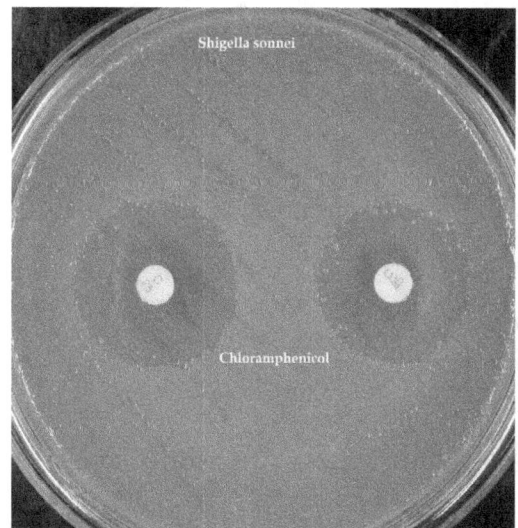
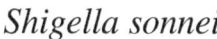

Shigella sonnei

Proteus vulgaris

Positive Control:

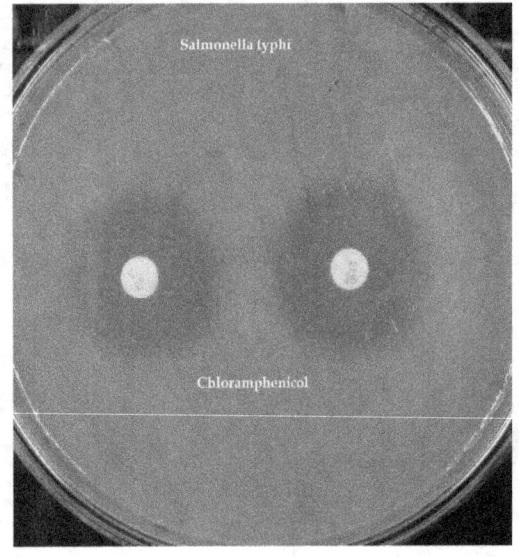
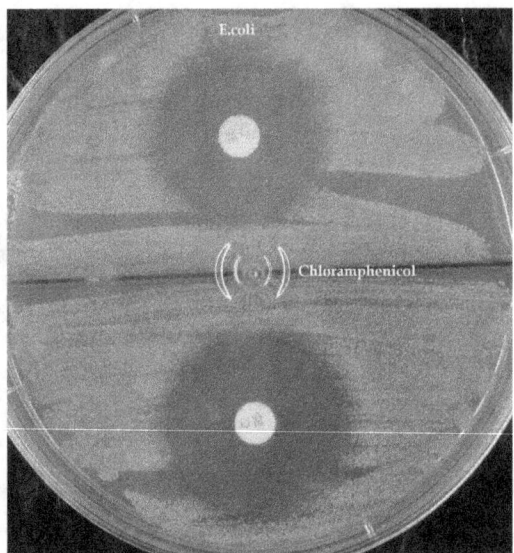

Salmonella typhi   *E.coli*

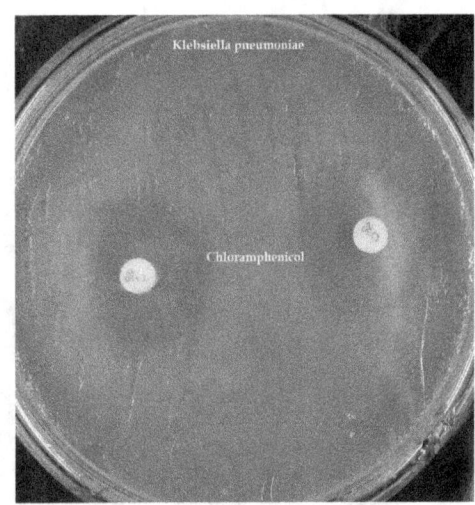

Klebsiella pneumonie

PART - III

DISCUSSION

Plants are important source of potentially useful structures for the development of new chemotherapeutic agents. The first step towards this goal is the *in vitro* antibacterial activity assay.[101] Crude plant extracts are generally a mixture of active and non-active compounds. A number of medicinal plants described in Unani System of Medicine still need to be testify according to the modern parameters to ensure their activity and efficacy. Many reports are available on the antibacterial, antifungal and anti-inflammatory properties of plants.[102, 103, 104, 105] Some of these observations have helped in identifying the active principle responsible for such activities and in the developing drugs for the therapeutic use in human beings.

In India, mortality rate due to infections is largely due to *S.aureus, Ps. aeruginosa, K.pneumonia, E.coli, P.vulgaris, S.sonnie, S.typhi, S. Paratyphi.*[106] The treatment and management of infections caused by these strains has become very difficult, because day to day increasing resistance to the available antibiotics, causes the challenge to discover newer and potent drugs is ever increasing. Therefore, studies were undertaken to test the extracts of Tukhm-e-Mooli against these pathogens. The highest activity was observed in Ethanolic and Methanolic extracts followed by Ethyl acetate, chloroform, Benzene, aqueous hot and aqueous cold.

The highest zone of inhibition (ZOI) in Ethanolic extract in *Pseudomonas aeruginosa* is 21.3±6.6 and lowest ZOI in *Salmonella paratyphi* is 13.3±1.5. In Methanolic extract the highest ZOI in *Proteus vulgaris* is 19.5±0.7 and lowest ZOI in *E. coli* is 12.5±0.7.

The zone of inhibition (ZOI) in ethyl acetate extract in *Proteus vulgaris* is 22.5±4.9, which is more than the zone of inhibition (ZOI) of standard drug chloramphenicol (20±0.5), and less than the zone of inhibition (ZOI) of standard drug ciprofloxacin (30±0.4)

Against *Pseudomonas aeruginosa* the zone of inhibition in ethanol, methanol. ethyl acetate, chloroform, aqueous hot and aqueous cold are respectively 21.3±6.6, 14.6±2.3, 18±0.5, 18.3±3.5, 13.3±2.0 and 9.3±0.5, which are more than the zone of inhibition (ZOI) of standard drug chloramphenicol (9±0.5), and less than the zone of inhibition (ZOI) of standard drug ciprofloxacin (30±0.4).

Against *staphylococcus aureus* the standard drug chloramphenicol has got resistance whereas the test drug shows sensitivity.

The zone of inhibition (ZOI) in Methanolic extract in *Salmonella paratyphi* is 14.6±1.5, which is more than the zone of inhibition (ZOI) of standard drug chloramphenicol (14±0.4), and less than the zone of inhibition (ZOI) of standard drug ciprofloxacin (30±0.5)

93

The highest antibacterial effect of Methanol and Ethanol extract against these organisms may be due to the ability of the Ethanol and Methanol to extract some of the active properties of these plants like Flavonoids, phenolic compounds, Saponins and other secondary metabolites which are reported as an antibacterial agents.[9] Flavonoids are found to be effective antimicrobial substances against a wide range of microorganisms, probably due to their ability to complex with extra cellular and soluble proteins and to complex with bacterial cell wall; more lipophilic Flavonoids may also disrupt microbial membrane. [107] Phenol and polyphenols present in the plants are known to be toxic to micro-organism. [108] Antibacterial activity of tannins may be related to their ability to inactivate microbial adhesins, enzymes and cell envelope transport proteins, they also complex with polysaccharides.[109]The antibacterial activity exhibited by *R. sativus* may be attributed to the various active constituents presents in it which either due to their individual or combined action.

Thus, the study ascertains the value of Tukhm-e-Mooli (*R. Sativus* L.) used in Unani System of Medicine. This could be of considerable interest to the development of new drugs.

CONCLUSION

The Unani drug Mooli (*Raphanus sativus* L.) of Brassicaceae family is an annual herb, cultivated all over sub-continent up to 16,000 ft in temperate and warm countries.[15] This drug is reputed medicine for urinary complaints, piles and gastrodynic pain.[15,16,17]

The present study shows that the Ethanolic and Methanolic extracts of the Tukhm-e-Mooli shows good antibacterial potentiality against all eight strains of pathogenic bacteria, used in this study. The test drug shows better activity than standard drug chloramphenicol against *Proteus vulgaris, Pseudomonas aeruginosa, Staphylococcus aureus and Salmonella paratyphi*, and shows less activity than ciprofloxacin.

The phytochemical analysis of Tukhm-e-Mooli shows the presence of different secondary metabolites or phytochemicals such as Alkaloids, Flavonoids, Glycosides, Carbohydrates, Phenol, Saponin, Sterol, Tannins and Protein. The antibacterial activity exhibited by Tukhm-e-Mooli may be attributed to these phytochemicals in it which either individual or combined action. Therefore, the results of present study provide a scientific validation of Unani Drug Tukhm-e-Mooli as an antibacterial agent. However, more investigations are needed in this direction before its clinical use.

SUMMARY

- The main aim of this study is to investigate the Antibacterial activity of Tukhm-e-Mooli.

- Review of both Unani and modern literature of Ilmul Jarasim (microbiology) has been done.

- Brief description of bacteria and bacteria used in experiment has mentioned.

- Review of Unani and botanical literature of Mooli has mentioned.

- Reviewed the research carried out on Mooli.

- Evaluation of Antibacterial activity has done.

- Phytochemical analysis of Tukhm-e-Mooli has done.

- Observations and result mentioned in Part-II

- Tukhm-e-Mooli shows significant Antibacterial potentiality.

Bibliography

BIBLIOGHRAPHY

1- Iwu, M.M., Duncan, A.R., Okunji, C.O., 1999: New Antimicrobials of plant origin. In: Perspective on New Crops and New uses. Ed: Janick, J., ASHS Press, Alexandria, VA, pg.457.

2- WHO Global Strategy for containment of antimicrobial resistance www.who.int/eme-documents/antimicrobial_resistance/docs/E Global_start.pdf

3- Reddy O.V.S., M. Manjunath, P.V.O.G., K.Sharma. *Invitro* Evaluation of antibacterial activity of *Actiniopteris Radiata* (Sw) Link. J. Pharmacy and Chemistry. Vol-2. Issue 2, pg.112-117.

4- Sabahat Saeed and P.Tariq. Effect of Some Seasonal Vegetables and Fruits on the growth of Bactria. Pakistan Journal of Biological Science 9(8): 2006 pg.1547-1551.

5- Overcoming microbial resistance http://www.who.int/infectious-disease-report/2000

6- Archibald L., Philips L,. Monnet D., Mc Gowan JE Jr, Tenover F,Gaynes R. Clin. Infect. Dis 1997; 24, pg.211-215.

7- Nascimento, G.G.F., J. Locatelli, P.C.Freitas and G.L. Silva 2000. Antibacterial activity of plant extracts and phytochemicals on antibiotics-resistant bacteria. Braz.J.Microbiol, 31, pg.247-256.

8- Tanaka, J.C.A., C.C. DeSilva, A.J.B. De Oliveira, C.V. Nakamura and B.P.D. Filho, 2006. Antibacterial activity of Indol alkaloids from Aspidosperma ramiflorum. Braz.J.Med. boil.Res. 39, pg.387-391.

9- Cowan, M.M., 1999. Plant products as antimicrobial agent. Clin. Microbiol. Rev., 12,pg. 564-582.

10- Press, J.B., 1996: Biodiversity: exciting prospects for drugs discovery and development. Meeting report of the Monroe Wall Symposium. Chemtracts-Organic chemistry 9, pg.286-298.

11- Eloff, J.N. 1998 (a): Which extract should be used for the screening and isolation of antimicrobial components from plants? Journal of Ethno pharmacology 60, pg. 1-8.

12- Bandow JE, Brotz H, Leichert LIO, Labischinski H and Hecker M. Proteomaic approach to understanding antibiotic action. Amicro. Agent. Chemother., 2003; 47, pg.948-955.

13- Rehman S, A Latif, S. Ahmad and A. U. Khan. Antibacterial activity of Shahtra (*Fumaria afficinales Linn.*) extracts against MRSA (Methicillin Resistant *Staphylococcus aureus*) Unani Medicus 2010 1(1), pg.57-61.

14- Stein, A.C., Sortino M., Avancini, C., Zacchino, S., Von Poser G., 2005: Ethnoveterinary medicine in the search for antimicrobial agents: Antifungal activity of some spacies of *Pterocaulon* (Asteraceae). Journal of Ethnopharmacology 99, pg. 211-214.

15- Kritikar, R.K. and B.D. Basu, 1987. Indian medicinal Plants. Vol-I Ed.2nd, India: International Book Distributors, 9/B, Rajpur Road, Dehradun, pg: 178.

16- A.A. Bin Sina, AL-QANUN FI´-TIB. Book II, Institute of History of Medicine and Medical research, New Delhi, 1987, pg.300.

17- Kabiruddin, Makhzanul Mufradat, Ejaz Publishing house New Delhi, p.558.

18- Chopra, R.N., S.L Nayar, and I.C. Chopra.1986 Glossary of Indian Medicinal plants (Including the supplements) Council of Scientific and Industrial Research, New Delhi. pg.85.

19- Ahmad S.I.,Introduction of Al-Umoor Al-Tabaiya, I[st] Edition,1980, Saini Printers Pahari Dhiraj, Delhi-6,pg.136.

20- Qadir A. Tarikh-e-Tibb wa Akhlaqiyat, Edition 2005, Rabbani Printers.New Delhi-6 pg.154.

21- Kasule,O.H. Achievements of The Muslim Civilization with Special Emphasis on Medicine.

(www.omerkasule.tripod.com & www.waljamaa.org/index.php)

22- Ibn Sina,Al Qanoon fil Tib Vol-IV, published by Idara kitab-us-shifa,New Delhi,2007,pg.87

23- IbnSina,Hummiyat-e-Qanoon, Idara kitab-us-shifa,New Delhi,2007,pg.144

24- Kabeeruddin,Armughan,DafterMaseeh,BazarNorulUmra,Hyderabad Deccan,1952,pg. 37-38.

25- Kabeeruddin, Resalah-e-Jarasim aur Tibb-e-Qadim, Dafter Maseeh, Bazar NorulUmra, Hyderabad Deccan, 1952, pg. 18.

26- Ibrahim S.B., The Islamic Medicine: 1000 years ahead of its times, (www.ishm.net/ishim/2/01.pdf)

27- www.muslimtent.com

28- www.theguardians.com/microbiology/gm_mbi01

29- www.bionewsonline.com/pub/pub1.htm

30- Ananthanarayan R. & Paniker C.K.J., Text book of Microbiology 8th Edition, University Press (India) Pvt. limited 2009, ISBN: 978-81-7371-6744, pg.3-8, 11-26,271,280,283-285, 288-300,315-316.

31- Madigon M., John M., Martinko J.(editors) 2000, Brock Biology of Microorganism 9th Edition, Prentice Hall India Pvt. Ltd, New Delhi, ISBN: 0-13-081922-0. pg. 17-28,102.

32- Arora D.R., Arora B., Text Book of Microbiology 3rd Edition CBS Publishers & distributers New Delhi 2008 ISBN: 978-81-239-1549-4. pg. 3-10, 13-26, 45, 348, 355, 362, 368, 375, 418.

33- Prohit S. S., Microbiology Fundamentals and Application 6th Edition 2003, Published by Student edition Jodhpur, ISBN: 81-88826-01-4, pg. 3-14, 37-53, 140-155, 540.

34- GodkerP. B., Text book of Medical Laboratory Technology, Edition 1994, Bhulani Publishing House, Dader Bombay, ISBN: 81-85578-10-9 pg. 283,348-361.

35- Belly A. Forbes, Daniel F. Sahm, Alice S. Weissfeld. Baily & Scott's Diagnostic Microbiology, 12th Edition 2007, Mosby Elsevier, Missouri-63146 ISBN:13:978-0-8089-2364-0, pg. 2-3, 17, 21, 194, 254, 323-326, 340.

36- Levinson W., E., Jawetz E., Medical Microbiology & Immunology, 3rd Edition, 1994, Prentice Hall India Pvt. Ltd, New Delhi ISBN: 0-8385-6221-3 pg. 13-14, 68-69, 91-102.

37- www.wikipedia.org

38- Todar K., PhD, Todler's Online text Book of Bacteriology

(http://textbookofbacteriolgy.net)

39- http://microbewiki.kenyon.edu

40- Collee J., G., A.G. Fraser, B.P. Marmion, A. Simmons.Mackie & Mc Cartney Practical Medical Microbiology. 2006 (Indian print) Published by Elsevier, a division of Reed Elsevier Indian Pvt. Limited, New Delhi-110065, ISBN: 978-81-312-0393-4, pg. 246, 363,368, 372, 385, 405, 413.

41- Green Wood D., R.C.B. Slack, J.F. Peutherer, Medical Microbilogy 16th Edition, 2006, (Indian print) Published by Elsevier, a division of Reed Elsevier Indian Pvt. Limited, New Delhi-110065, ISBN: 978-81-312-0100-8,pg.25-35,168,250,260,265,275,279,282.

42- Fyhrquist, P., Haeggstrom, C.A.,Vuorela, P., Hiltunen,R. (2007). Traditional medicinal uses and biological activities of some plant extracts of African *Combretum Loefl.*, *Terminalia* L. and *Pteleopsis* Engl. species (Combretaceae) Academic dissertation, University of Helsinki, ISBN 978-952-10-4057-3, pg.33-36.

43- Alanis, A. L., 2005: Resistance to Antibiotics: Are we in the Post-Antibiotic Era? Archives of Medical Research 36, pg.697-705.

44- Madigan, T. M., Martinko, J. M., Parker, J., 2000: Biology of Microorganisms, Ninth Edition,pg. 991.

45- Nikaido, H. 1996: Outer membrane, In: F. C. Neidhardt, R. Curtiss III, J. L. Ingraham, E. C. C. Lin,K. B. Low, Jr., B. Magasanik, W. S. Reznikoff, M. Riley, M. Schaechter, H. M. Umbarger (ed.),*Escherichia* coli and *Salmonella*; cellular and molecular biology, 2nd ed. American Society forMicrobiology, Washington D.C., pg.29-47.

46- Van Etten, H. D. et al., 1994: Two classes of plant antibiotics: phytoalexins versus phytoanticipins. *Plant Cell* 6, pg.1191-1192.

47- Schultes, R. E., 1978: The kingdom of plants, p. 208. In: W. A. R. Thomson (Ed.). Medicines from the Earth. McGraw-Hill Book Co., New York, N. Y.

48- Bailey, J. A., Mansfield, J. W., (eds.), 1982: Phytoalexins. Glasgow, Blackie. Pg.334.

49- Dixon, R. A., 1986: The phytoalexin response: elicitation, signaling and control of host gene expression. *Biol. Rev.* 61, pg.239-291.

50- Grayer, R. J., Harborne, J. B., 1994: A survey of antifungal compounds from plants, 1982-1993. *Phytochemistry* 37, pg. 19-42.

51- Osbourn, A. E., 1996: Preformed antimicrobial compounds and plant defense against fungal attack. *The Plant Cell* 8, pg. 1821-1831.

52- McMurchy, R. A., Higgins, V. J., 1984: Trifolirhizin and maackiain in red clover: Changes in *Fusariumroseum* "Avenaceum"-infected roots and *in vitro* effects on the pathogen. *Physiol. Plant. Pathol.* 25:229-238.

53- Higgins, V. J., Smith, D. G., 1972: Separation and identification of two pterocarpanoid phytoalexins produced by red clover leaves. *Phytopathology* 62,pg. 235-238.

54- Integrated Taxonomic Information System (ITIS). 1999b. *Raphanus sativus* L.ITISTaxonomicSerialNo.23290.RetrievedJuly21,2008. (http://www.itis.gov/)

55- http://plants.usda.gov/java/profile?symbol=RASA2

56- http://www.newworldencyclopedia.org/entry/Radish

57- Anonymous, The Wealth Of India, Vol-III, Edition 1985, Publication & Information Directorate, CSIR, Hill side road, New Delhi-12, ISBN:81-85038-00-7,pg. 366-372.

58- Anonymous, The Unani Pharmacopoeia of India, Part-I, Vol-V, 2010 CCRUM, Dept. Of AYUSH, Ministry of Health & Family Welfare Govt. Of India, New Delhi, pg.101.

59- Pullaiah T., Encyclopaedia of World Medicinal Plants, Vol-IV, 2006, Regency Publication New Delhi-8, ISBN: 81-89233-42-4, pg.1657-1658.

60- Khare C.P., Indian Medicinal Plants, 2007, Springer (India) Private Limited New Delhi-1 ISBN: 978-81-8128-658-1, pg.537.

61- Khory R. N., Katrak N.N., Materia Medica of India & Their therapeutics, 1981, Neeraj Publishing House New Delhi-52, pg.63.

62- F.L.S. Umberto Quattrocchi, CRC World Dictionary of Plant Names Vol-IV R-Z, 2000, CRC Press LLC,2000 Corporate Blvd., N.W., Boca Raton, Florida 33431, ISBN: 0-8493-2678-8 pg.2270.

63- Agharkar S.P., Medicinal Plants of Bombay Presidency, 1991, Scientific Publication Jodhpur-342001, ISBN: 81-7233-07-0, pg. 179-180.

64- Patil D.A., Herbal Cures Traditional approach, 2008, Aavishkar Publishers, Distributors, Jaipur-302003 Rajasthan India, ISBN: 978-81-7910-250-3, pg.176.

65- Vardhana R., Direct uses of Medicinal Plants and Their Identification, I[st] Edition 2008, Sarup & Sons New Delhi, ISBN: 81-7625-833-4, pg. 297.

66- Baldwin T., Seelzo V., Encyclopaedia of Natura Medica,Vol-III, 2008, Dominant Publishers & Distributers, New Delhi-51, ISBN: 81-7888-567-0, pg. 823.

67- Hooker J. D., Flora of British India Vol-I 1978, Periodical Expert Book Agency Delhi-32, pg.166.

68- Trivedi P.C., Indian Medicinal Plants, 2009, Aavishkar Publishers, Distributors, Jaipur-302003 Rajasthan India, ISBN: 978-81-7910-278-7, pg. 221, 269, 299.

69- Anonymous, Indian Medicinal Plants, Vol-IV, 1995, Orient Longman Limited Hyderabad-29, ISBN: 81-250-03037, pg.407-408.

70- Singh V., Pandey R.P., Ethanobotany of Rajasthan, India, 1998, Scientific Publishers Jodhpur, India P.O. Box no. 91, ISBN: 81-7233-182-7, pg.180.

71- Zohary D., Hopf M., Domestication of plants in the Old World, third edition (Oxford: University Press, 2000), pg.139.

72- Jain S.K., Dictionary of Indian folk medicine and Ethanobotany, 1991, Deep Publication Delhi-63, ISBN: 81-85622-00-0, pg.153.

73- Nadkarni A.K., Indian Materia Medica Vol-I, 2005, Bombay Popular Prakashan, Pvt. Ltd. Mumbai-34, ISBN: 81-7154-142-9, pg.1049-1050.

74- Rifat-uz-zaman, study of cardioprotective activity of *Raphanus sativus* L. in rabbits, Pakistani journal of Biological science 7 (5), 2004, ISSN: 1028-8880, pg.843-847.

75- Anwar R., Ahmad M., study of *Raphanus sativus* L. as hepatoprotective agent, journal of Ethnopharmacology Vol-68, Issues 1-3, 15 december 1999, pg. 335-338.

76- Al-QasoumiS.,Al-YahyaM.,Al-Hawiriny   T.,   Rafatullah   S., Gastroprotective effect of *Raphanus sativus* L. on experimental rat, FARMACIA 2008, Vol-LVI, 2 pg. 204.

77- Vargas S.R., Prez G.R.M., Zavala S.M.A., Antiurolithiatic activity of *Raphanus sativus* L. aqueous extract on rats, journal of Ethnopharmacology Vol-95, Issues 2-3, December 2004 pg. 169-172.

78- Tariq N. A., Tajulmufradat, 2004, Idara Kitab-ul-shifa, New Delhi-2, pg. 707-708.

79- Haleem A. M., Bustanulmufradat, 2002, Idara Kitab-ul-shifa, New Delhi-2, pg.563.

80- Ludhyanawi A., Ganjina-e-Tabib, 2000, Idara Kitab-ul-shifa, New Delhi-2, pg. 135.

81- ChughtaiG.M.M.,Chughtai F., Rahnuma-e-Aqaqeer Vol-I, Aejaz Publishing House New Delhi-2, pg. 486-491.

82- Baghdadi I. H., Kitab-al-Mukhtarat fil Tibb, Vol-II, 2005, CCRUM, New Delhi-58, pg. 237-238.

83- Ghani N., Khaza-nul-Advia part-I, 2009, Idara Kitab-ul-shifa, New Delhi-2, pg.1274-1276.

84- Ibn Sinna, Al-Qanoon fil-Tib Part-II, 2007, Idara Kitab-ul-shifa, New Delhi-2, pg.184.

85- Ibn Betar, Al-Jamiyat-ul-mufradat Al-Advia –Vol-III, 1999, CCRUM, New Delhi-58, pg.355-358.

86- http://www.druginfosys.com/herbal/Herb.aspx?Code=211&name=Raph anus%20sativus%

87- Rastogi R. P., Mehrotra B.N., Compodium of Indian Medicinal Plant Vol-I, 1995, Central Drug Research Institute Lucknow, Publication and Information Directorate, New Delhi, pg. 337.

88- Rastogi R. P., Mehrotra B.N., Compodium of Indian Medicinal Plant Vol-III, 1993, Central Drug Research Institute Lucknow, Publication and Information Directorate, New Delhi, ISBN: 81-85042-11-X, pg. 545.

89- Rastogi R. P., Mehrotra B.N., Compodium of Indian Medicinal Plant Vol-IV, 1995, Central Drug Research Institute Lucknow, Publication and Information Directorate, New Delhi, ISBN: 81-85042-13-6, pg. 621.

90- Duke J.A., Hand Book of Phytochemical Constituents of GRAS herbs and other economic plant, pg. 418. (www.ars-grin.gov/duke/farmacy2.pl)

91- Kabeeruddin, Byaz-e-Kabeer Vol-II, 2010, Idara Kitab-ul-shifa, New Delhi-2, pg.89, 146, 169, 178, 193, 333-334.

92- Anonymous, Qarabadin-e-Majeedi, 1986, Al India Unani Tibbi Conference, Delhi, Ajanta Offset and Packaging Limited, Delhi-52, pg. 153, 254, 320, 352, 384.

93- Rahman S.Z., Kitab-ul-Murakkbat, 1991, Publication Division Aligarh Muslim University, Aligarh, pg. 144, 169.

94- Anonymous, Unani Pharmacopoea of Andhra Pradesh Govt.Vol-I (Qarabadin-e-Sarkari), 1967, Dept. of Indian Medicine (AYUSH), Govt. Central Press, Hyderabad, pg.46.

95- Anonymous, Physiochemical standards of Unani formulations Part-3, 1993, Central council for research in Unani Medicine (CCRUM) Publication No.31 pg. A57-A60.

96- Evans WC in Trease and Evans, Pharmacognosy, 13th Edn. Bailliere Tindall. London, 1989, pg. 829-830.

97- Harborne JB. Phytochemical Methods, A guide to modern techniques of plant analysis, 3rd Edn. Chapman and Hall London 1998, pg. 302-312.

98- Reeves, D.S., 1989. Antibiotic assays, In: Howkey P.M., Levis, D.A.(Eds.), Medical Bacteriology, A practical Approach. IRL Press, Oxford, pg.195-221.

99- Lalitha, M.L., Manual on Antimicrobial Susceptibility testing (Under the Auspices of Indian Association of Medical Microbiology) pg.6-13.

100- Bhatt D. C. Ali A., Pharmaeutical Microbology Concept and Techniques, 2006, Birla Publications Pvt. Ldt. Delhi-32, ISBN: 81-86270-71-X, pg.119-124.

101- Tona, L., K. Kambu, N. Ngimbi, K. Cimanga and A.J. Vlietinck, 1998. Antiamoebic and phytochemical screening of some Congolese medicinal plants. J. Ethnopharmacol., 61,pg. 57-65.

102- Parekh, J. and S. Chanda, 2007b. Antibacterial and phytochemical studies on twelve species of Indian medicinal plants. African Journal of Biology Res., 10: 175-181.

103- Aliero, A.A. and A.J. Afolayan, 2006. Antimicrobial activity of Solanum tomentosum. African Journal of Biotechnology, 5,pg. 369-372.

104- Samy, R.P. and S. Ignacimuthu, 2000. Antibacterial activity of some folklore medicinal plants used by tribals in Western Ghats in India. J. Ethnopharmacol., 69,pg. 63-71.

105- Behera, S.K. and M.K. Misra, 2005. Indigenous phytotherapy for genito-urinary diseases used by the Kandha tribe of Orissa, India. J. Ethnopharmacol., 102, pg.319-325.

106- Muktanjali Arya, Prafull K Arya, Indian J Pathol.Microbiol 2005; 48, pg.266-269.

107- Tsuchiya, H., Sato, M., Miyazaki, T., Fujiwara, S., Tanigaki, S., Ohyama, M., Tanaka, T. and Iinuma M. J. Ethnopharmacol 1996; 50, pg. 27-34.

108- Mason, T.L. and Wasserman, B.P Phytochem 1987; 26, pg. 2197-2202.

109- Ya, C., Gaffney, S.H., Lilley, T.H. and Haslam, E. Carbohydrate polyphenol complexation. In Hemingway, R.W. and Karchesy J.J., Eds., Chemistry and Significance of Condensed Tannins, Plenum Press, New York. 1998, pg.552-553.

110- Anonymous, The Ayurvedic Pharmacopoeia of India Part-1 vol -3, 2008, CCRAM, Dept. Of AYUSH, Ministry of Health & Family Welfare Govt. Of India, New Delhi, pg.90. ISBN -81-901151-2-X, pg.110.

111- Perez Gutierrez, R.M. and Perez, R.L. (2004) *Raphanus sativus* (Radish): their chemistry and biology, The Scientific World JOURNAL **4**, pg.811-837.

www.ingramcontent.com/pod-product-compliance
Lightning Source LLC
Chambersburg PA
CBHW080820180526
45168CB00006B/2521